WOMEN AND MENTAL HEALTH

CHALLENGING
THE STEREOTYPES

Marian Barnes
and
Norma Anderson Maple

Published by
VENTURE PRESS
16 Kent Street
Birmingham
B5 6RD
Tel: 021 622 3911

First Published 1992

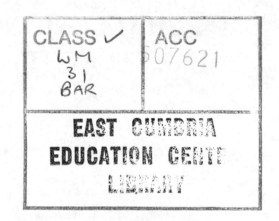

British Library Cataloguing in Publication Data

Women and Mental Health: Challenging
the Stereotypes
I. Barnes, Marian. II. Maple, Norma Anderson
362. 2082

ISBN 0 900102 85 3 (paperback)

CONTENTS

ACKNOWLEDGEMENTS

With acknowledgements and our thanks to the women who shared their experiences, both personal and professional, with us; to the women and men who found references and loaned us their books; and most especially to our partners, families and friends for their support.

1. WOMEN AND THE MENTAL HEALTH SYSTEM

Introduction

The origins of this book lie in experience of mental health social work practice, research into that practice, and in feminist theory. All three influences have convinced us that gender is a vital factor in understanding the experience of mental distress and mental disorder, and in finding ways to help those whose lives are affected by it. We feel that feminism both as a body of knowledge and as a different way of thinking about the world has much to offer mental health workers in this area.

We do not offer this perspective as an exclusive way of thinking about mental disorder. The issue is a highly complex one which we feel can only be understood by drawing on many types of knowledge and understanding, including the knowledge of the women and men whose lives are made more difficult by the experience of severe mental distress or disturbance. We do not want to reject the contribution of medicine either in diagnosis or treatment, nor to suggest that those who find drugs helpful in relieving the symptoms of their disorder are demonstrating a false consciousness. But we do want to challenge the pre-eminence of medicine in understanding the origins of mental distress and in controlling ways in which those experiencing such distress can be helped.

In addressing workers from various settings and disciplines, whose skills lie in helping people at the point of interaction between their personal and social lives, we think the feminist perspective has a particular relevance, but has not been given sufficient attention. Mental health workers are based in many different organisational settings. Some are professionally qualified, others are not. In many service settings multi-disciplinary mental health work is considered to provide most benefit to those experiencing mental distress. Whilst certain doctors and social workers have particular responsibilities in law (social workers approved under the 1983 Mental Health Act), other responsibilities for working with people in mental distress may be shared between social workers, counsellors, community psychiatric nurses and day centre or residential workers. Although our starting point has been social work, much of what we write in this book has direct relevance for other mental health workers. This is particularly significant at a time at which the organisation and location of mental health work are undergoing substantial change. We return to a discussion of this in the final chapter.

Whilst we have not examined the medical literature, in the (very few) standard social work texts which deal specifically with mental health social work, there are few direct references to the different ways in which men and women may experience mental distress, nor how they may need to influence social work practice. Alan Butler and Colin Pritchard, for example in 'Social Work and Mental Illness' (Butler and Pritchard, 1983) acknowledge in their opening chapter that there should be a willingness to look at the wider social context in which the unusual or disturbing behaviour defined as evidence of mental illness takes place. However, they make no reference to the relevance of gender in this context. They also only very occasionally recognize that both social workers and those who become social work clients may be women.

Such 'gender blindness' is largely shared by Barbara Hudson in 'Social Work with Psychiatric Patients' (Hudson, 1982). She does on occasion recognise that there is a difference in the extent to which different forms of mental disorder are experienced or identified amongst men and women, but she does not explore the reasons for this in any detail. An exception is Alison Corob's book 'Working with Depressed Women' (Corob, 1987), which provides an important alternative view of mental health social work, but as its title implies its focus is specifically on depression.

The lack of attention given to the significance of gender in mental health social work is symptomatic of the invisibility of gender issues in social work generally. As Brook and Davis (1985) note:

> 'The significance and consequences of the predominance of women in the day to day negotiations between social workers, clients and their families have not been explicitly discussed. Most social work literature has taken for granted that this is a normal, and therefore unimportant, fact of professional life.' (p.5)

A secondary purpose of this book is to try to use a different language to describe the experiences of women who may come into contact with social workers because of their mental health problems.

In doing so we will draw on ways in which women have talked to us about their experiences. One of the features of the dominance of medical ideology and bureaucracy in mental health has been that psychiatric language is used not only by psychiatrists, but also by others who are trying to describe and understand mental disorder. The result of this is that terms describing psychiatric diagnoses are often used inaccurately by other professionals. Such terms have also entered day to day language as terms of abuse or as a casual and demeaning way of describing unusual or unfamiliar behaviour.

Many of those to whom psychiatric labels have been applied reject these not only because of the stigma which attaches to them, but also because they have no meaning to them and totally fail to describe the personal experiences involved. Being 'ill' may be more socially acceptable than being 'mad', but the term schizophrenia has become almost synonymous with madness so that it is uncertain that it is any the less stigmatising. Many mental health professionals themselves also recognise that these labels can be not only inaccurate but also determine how people are responded to, often over the course of many years.

We need to make a few more introductory comments about our subject. Firstly, a discussion which takes gender as a starting point must reflect on certain comparisons between men and women. Assumptions about what is 'normal' and appropriate behaviour for women and men can cause stress for men who do not perceive themselves as having stereotypical masculine attributes. The significance of gender for an analysis of men's mental health is undeveloped if not non-existent. But we leave that for male colleagues to follow up! However, we do hope that our readers will include men as well as women because if feminism is to have a creative impact on mental health practice and on the organizations in which that practice is carried out, it must influence the practice of men as well as women.

Secondly, our discussions relate primarily to the experiences of white women in western society. The experiences of black women living in the United Kingdom will be affected by cultural differences, racism and in some cases language difficulties as well as by sexism. The experience of sexism is different in different cultures. We would not wish to ignore the mental health problems of black women and we will refer to the experience of black women in this book. But we do not feel that as two white women we can provide a complete understanding or analysis of the particular problems of black women, and again we hope that others may take this up.

We will not be able to consider all the specific experiences which contribute to mental health difficulties of women in different circumstances. This is not a comprehensive textbook and we cannot provide sufficient case studies to demonstrate the particular difficulties experienced, for example, by lesbian women or women with disabilities. We acknowledge that the origins of mental health problems and the response received from mental health professionals will vary for women in different social classes and circumstances and we will consider some of the implications of this in talking of service and resource implications. A woman-centred practice cannot ignore the experiences which divide and separate women as well as unite them.

In this introductory chapter we will explore three issues which provide different types of evidence about the differences gender makes to the experience of mental distress. The first concerns the way in which mental health and mental ill health are defined; the second is evidence of the different rate at which mental disorder is apparently experienced by men and women and the different types of diagnoses that are applied to men and women; and the third is evidence of different professional responses once women and men have come into contact with the mental health system. In this discussion we will draw on research conducted in this area, including some in which we ourselves have been involved, and on conversations with women who have had experience of the mental health system. Quotes from women which are not referenced are taken from conversations which we have had whilst collecting material for this book.

These three issues are not entirely separate. Definitions affect the identification of mental disorder and hence the number of people who are considered to be 'mentally ill'. Professional responses have a considerable influence on what comes to be defined as mental disorder in a society in which mental distress has come to be primarily the province of doctors rather than lawyers or priests. But for the purposes of making sense of the evidence we will consider each separately.

Definitions of mental health and mental ill health

'Hysteria, n. Functional disturbance of nervous system
(esp. of women), characterised by anaesthesia, convul-
sions, etc., & usu. attended with disturbance of moral and
intellectual faculties (formerly thought to be due to disturbance of womb); morbid excitement.' (Concise Oxford
Dictionary, 1966.)

When men sent off in a patriotic fervour to fight for their country
in the First World War returned home experiencing 'shell shock'
and exhibiting the same symptoms of 'hysteria' which had been
identified to almost epidemic levels amongst women at the turn of
the century, it created a profound shock to the nation's perceptions
of 'manliness'. By definition men could not be hysterical and yet
here were thousands of young men exhibiting symptoms such as loss
of the sense of smell and taste, impaired vision, loss of memory,
impotence, continual weeping, an inability to move out of the foetal
position, without there being any evidence of a physiological cause
for such a lack of control over their physical and emotional
responses (see Showalter, 1987). Clearly 'disturbance of the womb'
was not the cause, but one response of psychiatrists at the time was
to suggest that the men so affected were certainly effeminate and
probably homosexual — a 'real man' could not possibly respond to
the horrors of war in that way.

The suggestion that mental disorder is more normally a
characteristic of women than it is of men has received confirmation
from a number of research studies which have set out to explore
perceptions of mental health and mental ill health. Such studies are
themselves grounded in studies of more general perceptions about
the differences between men and women. For example Rosenkrantz
and colleagues (Rosenkrantz *et al*, 1968) studied perceptions of
male and female characteristics and identified a number of
stereotypical characteristics. More of those characteristics defined
as 'socially desirable' were ascribed to men than to women. They
then looked at self-perceptions according to gender. It appeared that
both women and men were influenced by popular beliefs about the
nature of women and men, but could not entirely go along with such
beliefs as they applied to themselves. There was a discrepancy

between how they saw themselves and how they thought women or men were normally viewed.

But there is also evidence from similar studies which suggests that stereotypical beliefs work to maintain existing sex roles - 'is' becomes 'ought' as Fransella and Frost (1982) describe it. Hence, personal perceptions of self which do not coincide with what are considered to be the normal perceptions of what a woman should be are a potential source of difficulty. This is made worse by the fact that there appear to be socially desirable characteristics, particularly relating to competency, which women are not supposed to possess. Fransella and Frost conclude from their review of such studies:

> 'In our view, the stereotype is particularly disabling. Women are valued for a rather narrow set of personal qualities. Indeed, being valued for these particular qualities (some of which are desirable in themselves, and for men as well as women) may in itself be a problem. For women are supposed to restrict themselves to pursuing the 'feminine' virtues. Someone once said that sitting on a pedestal leaves you very little room for manoeuvre. There are qualities that can be regarded as vital for any individual who has found personal independence and responsibility. But these are the very qualities that women must avoid lest they be thought masculine'. (Fransella and Frost, 1982: 52.)

Mental health is not something that is easily defined. Studies which have tried to explore how people describe mentally healthy adults have demonstrated the extent to which such concepts are socially determined - there is no absolute definition of mentally healthy behaviour and characteristics:

> 'Jahoda (1958) emphasised such concepts as self-acceptance, integration of personality, autonomy, perception of reality and environmental mastery. Clearly, all such concepts are utterly dependent on social meaning and interpretation. When, for instance, does single-mindedness become an obsession, or personal autonomy become self-

aggrandisement? Whose reality must be correctly perceived before we are prepared to say that someone is in touch with it?' (Barnes, Bowl and Fisher, 1990: 11/12.)

Reality for a working class woman is likely to be round-the-clock responsibility for child care, making ends meet on an inadequate income, ensuring that her husband's sexual and emotional needs are met before hers are, and negotiating with teachers, the housing department and other representatives of officialdom. This is very different from the daily reality of a consultant psychiatrist in a high-status, well-paid job which affords him considerable power and respect, who returns to a comfortable home and a wife who has ensured that he has few domestic concerns to trouble him once he has stopped working. We accept the stereotypes contained in this description, but for the woman whose words we quote below, the different realities of her and her psychiatrist's world proved a gulf which could not be bridged:

> 'After the abuse incident, I went to see a psychodynamic psychiatrist, but he was so removed from reality that when I tried to explain about the money situation he just couldn't see that money could be a bar to me leaving. He was just so wrapped up in everybody's inner worlds rather than outer worlds it wasn't any good at all. Then we saw a behavioural psychologist for marital therapy and he was trying to get us to do things that would please the other partner, but I felt so negative towards him I didn't want to do anything that pleased him; so that was a washout as far as I was concerned' (quoted in Corob, 1987: 18).

If concepts of mental health are socially constructed, and if beliefs about both the actual and the desirable characteristics of men and women are different, then it is not surprising that ideas about what is a 'mentally healthy' woman differ from ideas about a mentally healthy man. Broverman and her colleagues (Broverman *et al*, 1970) found that the terms used by both male and female clinicians to describe healthy women added up to a very negative assessment and one that varied more from an assessment of ideal health than did the descriptions of a normal healthy man. For these clinicians, healthy women differed from healthy men by being more submissive, less independent, less adventurous, more easily influenced, less aggressive, less competitive, more excitable in minor crises, having their feelings more easily hurt, being more emotional, more conceited about their appearance and less objective.

Other research by Fabrikant (1974) confirmed that male therapists felt that the majority of female concepts were negative, whilst the majority of male concepts were positive, and later work by Jones and Cochrane (1981) indicated that such prejudices were not the sole preserve of the medical profession. They too identified a clear differentiation in the concepts chosen to describe a mentally ill man compared with those chosen to describe a 'normal' man. Yet there was much less difference in the descriptions of a 'normal' woman and a mentally ill woman.

One of the results of male dominance has been to ensure that, by definition, characteristics typically associated with women are not only less desirable, but also less healthy. The irrational, subjective woman by her very nature is closer to madness than the scientific, rational male who not only controls most of the external world, but also has greater control over his own physical and mental well-being.

> Whilst the name of the symbolic female disorder may change from one historical period to the next, the gender asymmetry of the representational tradition remains constant. Thus madness, even when experienced by men, is metaphorically and symbolically represented as feminine: a female malady. In French, for example, the man dressed as a woman, the drag queen, is even called 'the madwoman' — la folle. (Showalter, 1987: 4.)

But they want to have it both ways. Whilst women by their nature are seen to be closer to madness than are men, mental disorder amongst women is often identified by reference to behaviour which apparently deviates from what is regarded as proper feminine behaviour.

Two British sociologists have made an interesting comparison of their treatment for migraine. Whereas David Oldman, a family man with a high-powered job, never encountered any suggestion that his way of life was responsible for his attacks, Sally MacIntyre, as a single research student, was told that her migraine resulted from her not having a boyfriend and from her sublimation of her desire to have children (MacIntyre and Oldman, 1977: 62) (Dale and Foster, 1986).

Soldiers responding to seeing their friends blown to bits by retreating into muteness or breaking down into floods of tears 'for no reason', were considered to be effeminate. Women demonstrating the socially desirable male characteristics of assertiveness, competence and adventurousness which lead to rejection of a highly constrained role for themselves, are in danger of being labelled mentally disordered. Just as many of their sisters in a less conscious response to the mind-numbing tedium of their daily lives were labelled as hysterics in the late-nineteenth and early-twentieth centuries.

Both feminist and non-feminist writers have commented on the apparent anomaly in the comparison between mental disorder and other forms of 'deviance' when related to gender. Whilst women figure more frequently in the mental health statistics (see below), men outnumber women in recorded statistics for a wide range of deviant behaviour: alcoholism, drug abuse, crime, violence and suicide. Barrett and McIntosh (1982) conclude that this must in some way derive from gender differences in the relationship between private and public lives. Cochrane (1983) suggests that this has something to do with the way in which gender affects definitions of behaviour. Elsewhere one of us has suggested that 'It may be that men are being deprived of the potential benefits of mental health services because they themselves are less likely to identify their problems in terms of mental distress and to seek help for them on those terms. (Barnes, Bowl and Fisher, 1990: 133.)

Unravelling the relationship between the way in which behaviour is defined and identified cannot lead to the identification of cause and effect. But the comparison between mental disorder and criminality is an important one as it provides another perspective on the question of what is normal and what is abnormal behaviour for men and women. 'Boys will be boys', but if a woman deviates from accepted patterns of feminine behaviour she may be considered mad as well as bad.

Those deviations have often been given a specifically sexual connotation which has taken on a particular form of representation in tune with the culture of the time. Elaine Showalter has provided a vivid historical account of 'The Female Malady', but she suggests that the view of mental disorder amongst women being associated with both their emotionality and sexuality is not one which has been confined to history. This was confirmed to us in the following description of a young woman's encounter with a psychiatrist at a time in her life when she was trying to make sense of a disrupted family life which had included sexual abuse by a family friend:

> 'I did go to a psychiatrist because in the beginning you go along with this. You think, 'Oh a psychiatrist, that's got to be someone I can talk to!' The first psychiatrist I ever saw, I think the first question he asked me, apart from my name, was 'Do you have orgasms?' It was very much centred around my sex life (I didn't have one at the time), around whether my periods were regular. They decided I was suffering from pre-menstrual tension - I didn't know what that was then, and I took these tablets which made no difference.'

The association between mental disorder and physiological and behavioural aspects of women's sexuality often gives the impression of both an obsession with and fear of that sexuality amongst those empowered to define such disorder.

Are Women More Often Mentally Ill Than Men?

There is considerable evidence to show that women are more often identified as being mentally ill or as experiencing emotional problems which affect their ability to live happy and fulfilled lives than are men. This evidence relates to figures for hospital admissions (both voluntary and compulsory admissions), to referrals to general practitioners and to findings of general population surveys which have sought to identify the prevalence of mental health problems amongst the population at large. It is possible to suggest why this should be so by reference to the circumstances of women in a male-dominated society, but the previous discussion indicates that the question of what is defined as mental ill health is itself a function of that domination. The meaning of such evidence is therefore not as straightforward as it might appear.

Some figures are important to illustrate the basis for our concerns.We know that women are admitted to psychiatric hospital at a rate of 468 per 100,000 whilst the equivalent rate for men is 364 per 100,000 (DHSS, 1986). We know that women are more likely than are men to be referred to Approved Social Workers (ASWs) for assessment for admission under the Mental Health Act. During one year in which social workers in 42 Social Services Departments throughout England and Wales collected information women were referred at a rate of 82.5 per 100,000 whilst the equivalent rate was 68.4 per 100,000 in the case of men (Barnes, Bowl and Fisher, 1990). Women are more likely to be diagnosed as suffering from psychological problems by GPs (Goldberg and Huxley, 1980), they are twice as likely to be taking tranquillisers, and two-thirds of those taking anti-depressants are women (Curran and Golombok, 1985). Women also attend psychiatric hospitals as out-patients and as day patients in greater numbers than men, and they are more likely to be receiving domiciliary visits from psychiatrists (Cochrane, 1983). Amongst clients of social workers who may or may not be defined as 'mental health cases' women outnumber men quite considerably. In Fisher's *et al.* study of mental health social work, women outnumbered men by 2 to 1 in the cases studied (Fisher, Newton and Sainsbury, 1984).

If assumptions about what are mentally healthy characteristics put women at a disadvantage from the start, then it is not surprising that instruments designed to measure the extent of mental health problems amongst the population identify more women than men. Nor is it surprising that GPs, who are most often the first port of call for health problems, identify more of those problems as having a mental health component amongst their women patients than amongst their men patients.

Another factor which gets in the way of assuming an equation between the comparative levels of use of mental health services and the objective levels of experience of mental disorder, is that women are in general more likely to go to their G.P. when they have worries about their health than are men. Also they are more likely to identify their own problems as those of their emotional state than are men.

The reasons for women's predominance amongst users of mental health services have to be sought not only in the way in which behaviour comes to be defined as evidence of mental ill health but also in the social circumstances of women's lives. In order to start to understand what this means it is first of all important to look a bit more closely at the differences. Hospital admission rates are affected by age, by marital status and by diagnosis. Young men have a higher admission rate than young women, but women outnumber men in the middle-age and older-age groups. Amongst single, widowed and divorced people, the rate of admission to psychiatric hospital is higher for men than for women. But amongst married people the rate of admission is much higher for women than men and the predominance of married people in the adult population means that the overall rate of admission is higher amongst women than men (Cochrane, 1983). The number of men and women admitted to hospital with a diagnosis of schizophrenia is similar, but women are twice as likely to be admitted to hospital with a diagnosis of depressive psychosis or psychoneuroses.

The study of referrals to social workers for assessments under the Mental Health Act, 1983 referred to above found that the marital status and other circumstances of the men and women involved were often different:

'Overall women were more likely to be living in what is regarded as the normal circumstance for adults. They were more likely to be living with a partner of their own generation in accommodation which was personal to them. Men, on the other hand, were less likely to have broken away from their family of birth and less likely to have forged partnerships which led to the creation of new households of their own. This is partly to do with age - more of the men referred were young adults, whereas women were more often middle aged or elderly. But the fact remains that amongst those referred to social workers in need of assessment because of mental health problems, more women than men were in situations which would not normally be regarded as indicative of risk.' (Barnes, Bowl and Fisher, 1990: 139.)

The general conclusion must be that it is not simply the difference in biological sex which can account for the differences in the experience of emotional distress. This conclusion is reinforced by the fact that these observed gender differences are not universal. As Ray Cochrane concludes: 'It is difficult to see how a major biological difference between the two sexes in the susceptibility to mental illness could have appeared only recently, only in certain ethnic groups, and only in the married. Obviously any kind of biological explanation must be placed firmly in a social context for it to be able to provide a useful explanation for differences in mental illness.' (Cochrane, 1983 pp.45 - 6.)

George Brown and Tirril Harris undertook what has come to be regarded as a classic study of women and depression (Brown and Harris, 1978) in an attempt to define 'The Social Origins of Depression'. This study, of working class women in a part of London, took as its starting point the fact that depression is more often diagnosed amongst women than men and sought to explore what were the circumstances which appeared to be associated with depression amongst this group of women. They found that the women they studied were more likely to experience depression if certain 'predisposing factors' were present: they had three or more children under 14 living at home, they were unemployed, they had lost their mother in childhood, or they lacked an intimate confiding relationship.

We have no cause to doubt the validity of these findings which seem very understandable factors which could contribute to depression. However, what this study does not do is explore why such experiences should contribute to women's poor mental health. Men could have the same life experiences and may or may not experience depression as a result. A feminist analysis would not interpret these findings as evidence that women are less able to stand up to difficult life experiences, but would explore why it is that these common circumstances are apparently dangerous to women's mental health.

Another research project adopted a comparative approach in order to explore whether there is any evidence of a different rate of mental distress between men and women. Rachel Jenkins (Jenkins, 1985) designed a study which would first of all identify a group of men and women in the same social environment, of a similar age, level of occupation and subject to similar levels of stress and support. The group decided on were men and women between 20 and 35 years old, who were all direct entry civil servants of the executive officer grade working in the Home Office in London and who had been in post for less than 10 years. She compared their mental health by using the General Health Questionnaire in order to identify those who showed some evidence of mental health difficulties, then the Clinical Interview Schedule to explore these problems in more depth. There was no difference between men and women in the prevalence of mental health problems and no real difference in the severity of those problems. She concluded that the differences which have been identified in other studies and in the referral rates to mental health services are most likely to be due to environmental causes.

From the evidence that is available it is hard not to conclude that there are characteristics of 'normal' family life which are less supportive of women's mental health than of men's. Why should this be so? One woman who was attending a mental health centre in Bradford suggests one reason:

'I was taking on so much of the worry of all the family.
Our house was like the citizen's advice bureau. I wanted
to scream "Shut up! You are upsetting me", but the scream
stayed there; it wouldn't come out.' (Quoted in Bailey,
1987: 30.)

The problems of family life for women have been a focus for
much feminist analysis. In 'The Anti-Social Family' Michele
Barrett and Mary McIntosh (1982) discuss how family life is seen
to be a very private and protected set of relationships. This means
both that behaviour within its sphere is not open to criticism (it was
only as we were starting to write this book that it started to become
possible to claim rape within marriage) and that it should provide a
sufficient source of satisfying and intimate relationships. Yet men
through their work outside the home more often have a whole
different set of relationships and roles which are a potential source
of satisfaction. If women work outside the home it is more likely to
be through economic necessity and to be in low paid, less satisfying
forms of employment. Thus women are more dependent on good
quality family relationships than are men, but are also in a position
where it is they who are seen to be responsible for meeting the
emotional needs of the rest of the family. As Barrett and McIntosh
say:

'It would be simplistic also to see becoming mentally ill
just as a measure of suffering. Yet we do need to explain
why women who work outside the home and unmarried
women are less likely to become depressed than the
housebound wife. It is clear that being a housewife can
drive women mad, though why they tend so often to
experience depression and 'nerves', rather than, say,
anger or revolt is perhaps less clear.' (Barrett and McIntosh, 1982: 59.)

Feminist psychologists have sought to understand why the
quality of relationships may be more significant to women's
feelings of well-being than is apparently generally the case in
relation to men (Kaplan and Surrey, 1984). They have pointed to
the way traditional theories of development emphasise separation

and independence from others as signs of healthy adult development. Viewing oneself as a person in relation to others and thus seeing part of your identity as tied up with such relationships has tended to be seen as a sign of immaturity. What such theories deny is the positive aspects of mutuality and sensitivity to others and indeed the fact that 'the ability to experience, comprehend, and respond to the inner state of another person is a highly complex process relying on a high level of psychological development and ego strength' (Kaplan and Surrey, op.cit: 82).

The psychiatrist Jean Baker Miller wrote:

> 'Male society, by depriving women of the right to its major 'bounty' — that is, development according to the male model — overlooks the fact that women's development is proceeding but on another basis. One central feature is that women stay with, build on, and develop in a context of connections with others. Indeed, women's sense of self becomes very much organised around being able to make and then to maintain affiliations and relationships. Eventually for many women the threat of disruption of connections is perceived not as just a loss of a relationship but as something closer to a total loss of self.' (Miller, 1988: 83.)

Miller proposes that we need a different terminology for theories of development which does not discriminate against women.

In proposing an alternative theory of personal development which emphasises the 'self-in-relation' and collaborative modes of operating, one aim would be to promote a positive view of women's needs for high quality relationships rather than seeing this as a weakness. This aim is also seen to have potential positive outcomes for men as well. Gaining acceptance for a basic theory of personal development which does not discriminate against women from the start is a long-term goal. But social workers and others who aim to help women whose low self-esteem may be both cause and result of considerable mental health problems could well make use of such

16

ideas in their practice in order to persuade women that a need for 'intimate confiding relationships' is not a sign of over-dependency.

Doctors and Social Workers — Dealing with the 'experts'.

Inevitably in describing how women come to be identified as 'mentally ill' we have started to talk about the way in which they are treated when they come into contact with professionals in the mental health system. In this section we will focus on that in rather more detail.

> 'Most doctors are men, most patients are women. I have no doubt that there are some paternal, protective and sexual feelings between doctors and patients that make male doctors think they must help women more [than men]. I think that women are also under far more stress than men basically in a sexist society. It's also something to do with the way men present themselves. It is a sort of macho thing; they are less involving, more matter of fact: here's the problem and let's see what we can do about it. I feel that prescribing for men is not so urgent or so necessary. Men talk about problems in a different way. I suppose the one benefit of a macho approach to things is that they tend to say 'I don't need tablets, I can manage it myself'.' (General Practitioner quoted in Curran and Golombok, 1985)

This General Practitioner acknowledges a difference in the way he treats his men and women patients which derives from their gender rather than any objective difference in their medical or other needs. Men make it easy for him not to take responsibility for them, whilst fundamental assumptions about women's weakness and dependence result in a response (prescribing tranquillisers) which often results in increasing dependence both on him and the drugs he prescribes.

'GP bashing' is a popular sport amongst social workers, but are they entirely innocent when it comes to sexist responses to their clients? The following quote from a social work case file suggests not: 'Inadequate manipulative woman whose tendency to depression leads her to neglect her home and family. In spite of a supportive husband she does not seem able to function in her role as wife and mother although there has been no success in persuading her not to have more children.' (Quoted in Hale, 1983: 171.)

We do not know whether the social worker who wrote this was a man or woman and we would not want to suggest that it was inevitably a man. The point here is that the view being expressed is every bit as stereotyped as that implied in the General Practitioner's statement, and in fact has an added dimension of blame of the woman concerned.

Both such statements reflect an underlying power difference between the 'professional' and the 'client' or 'patient'. At times of difficulty or stress, when people cannot make sense of what is happening to them, or feel physically unable to deal with the complex range of responsibilities which are part of daily life, they may turn for help to someone professionally designated as a helper or healer. In some instances other people make that decision for them and they find themselves, whether they like it or not, on the receiving end of professional attention. Both situations put the recipient in a subordinate position which can be exploited by the professional concerned. Sometimes this can be a passive exploitation as in the case of this encounter between a young woman and a psychiatrist:

'He was one of these people who sat in a corner and didn't say a word. I sat and didn't say a word because I didn't know what to say. What I wanted was someone to lead me or ask a question . . . We had an hour like this, with me frantically trying to think of something I should say that would get a response from this person. I was sitting there feeling dreadful, frightened and totally inadequate because I wanted to get a response from him, to smile, say something. . . . I couldn't think of anything to say. . . . At the end of this meeting he then labelled me mild schizophrenic having not got any information from me, not asked me one question except to confirm my name. I went out of there thinking I'm not schizophrenic, that I do know.'

In other cases the potential for abuse of power is more blatant In America a study conducted in the early 1970s found that:

Approximately three times as many women as men have received psychosurgery. The claim that psychosurgery has sometimes been used on women primarily to push women into traditional caring roles is supported by the overt statements of certain psycho-surgeons, one of whom observed that after a lobotomy 'some women do the dishes better, are better housewives and comply with the sexual demands of their husbands . . . . It takes away their aggressiveness'. (Roth and Lerner, 1974, quoted in Dale and Foster, 1986.)

It must immediately be acknowledged that the Mental Health Act 1983 in this country defines strict rules for the use of psycho-surgery which should mean it is used only in extreme cases. But the point we want to make is that, within the career of psychiatrists who are currently practising, that type of attitude existed. Because the power wielded by them could result in irreversible treatments, the aim of which was the keeping of women in their 'rightful place'. A less extreme indication of this is the inclusion until fairly recently of 'Housewives' Syndrome' as an entry in psychiatric textbooks, and the fact that similar terminology can still be heard from psychiatrists in influential positions today.

The power of psychiatric professionals can be seen as one example of a general trend in which science and the primarily male professionals who have controlled it have moved in on territory previously occupied by those whose knowledge was based on experience, observation or religious lore. Often that development has been presented as one of progress from the dark ages of superstition into the clarity of scientific thought. Barbara Ehrenreich and Deirdre English present a rather different picture:

> 'The rise of the experts was not the inevitable triumph of right over wrong, fact over myth; it began with a bitter conflict which set women against men, class against class. Women did not learn to look to an external 'science' for guidance until after their own skills had been ripped away, and the 'wise women' who preserved them had been silenced, or killed.' (Ehrenreich and English, 1979: 33.)

Once healing had been something carried out by women both within their local communities and, in the case of the most skilled, wider afield. The healing skills were widely shared amongst women so that they had a network of information sharing and support and their knowledge was built up by the combined experience and wisdom of centuries of healers. Witch hunts were only one result of the fear and threat felt by men about these female skills.

One of the results of this general move towards the professionalisation of both healing and care has been that definitions of problems belong to the experts rather than to those experiencing the problem. If the expert definition is rejected, then the person is described as 'lacking insight' into their condition. Yet one result of medicine claiming expertise over that area of human experience labelled 'mental illness' has been that for those who are feeling stressed, unhappy, or depressed, or whose thoughts are disorganised so that it becomes difficult to control their lives, in some cases to the extent that it feels that outside forces are taking over, for people who are worried or frightened about what is happening to them, the only person they can think to turn to is their GP. The GP is very likely to define the problem as an illness, because if a woman is not ill why has she come to see him? The woman whose encounter with a psychiatrist we described above said that she was desperate for someone to talk to who would understand and help her work through her problems. She went to her GP who then sent her to the psychiatrist concerned and she came out of his office with a psychiatric diagnosis. If she had been a young man it is far less likely that referral to a psychiatrist would have been the outcome of the GP visit. Goldberg and Huxley (1980) found that young men were one of the groups least likely to be diagnosed by GPs as suffering from psychological as opposed to physical problems.

Once referred to a psychiatrist, the woman's experience will be affected by the needs of the medical bureaucracy as well as by the professional opinion of the 'expert' she meets. The psychiatric model requires that each patient receives a diagnosis. This is intended to assist in the development of the treatment strategy but is also used as a 'shorthand' way of describing someone's condition in medical discussion. It is also an administrative aid, and in a National Health Service based on internal markets, may affect resource allocation. In the United States, for example, the medical diagnosis is critical in whether the patient receives funding for 7 or 14 days' group therapy.

The discussion so far in this section has concentrated on the way in which the primarily male medical profession responds to women with mental health problems. We need to justify that in a book that addresses mental health work in a variety of disciplines and settings. In part it is simply a reflection of how little attention has been given to the way in which social workers and other mental health workers respond to people in general and women in particular whose mental health difficulties result in them becoming social work clients. The dominance of the medical profession in the care and treatment of those experiencing mental disorder provides the justification for our discussion for two reasons. Firstly, it means that women's experience of seeking help for their problems is likely to be coloured by their experience of medical responses. The medical definition of the nature of the problem may already be established and may have been accepted by the woman herself as an explanation of what is wrong with her. Acceptance by some clients of the 'illness model' was described by Sylvia Bailey in her study of a mental health centre:

> 'The referral to a mental health centre brought a welcome relief. Fifteen people thought they were ill in some way and there was a belief that they would be understood by the staff at Bolton Road. Many clients expressed the feeling that their bodies had failed them or were exhibiting signs that things were going wrong for them.' (Bailey,

1987.) Mental health workers need to be aware of the extent to which their clients may have accepted or rejected the explanations which have already been offered to them about their problems.

The second point concerns the relationship of social work to medicine. The divorce of psychiatric social work from health authority control after the establishment of social services departments was not popular with many psychiatrists. Before then, it was often the case that psychiatrists valued social workers to the extent that they could claim that they were 'my social workers'. Concern has been expressed in some quarters that not too much has changed over the years and there is a view that hospital social workers should not carry out the duties of Approved Social Workers because their independence from psychiatrists cannot be guaranteed. If social work, psychology, psychotherapy and psychiatric nursing are subservient to medicine in this field there is a danger that attitudes prevalent amongst medical practitioners will be adopted, either because of the belief that the attitudes of the dominant profession are right, or because, to gain acceptance, social workers and others feel they should not be too confrontational. Some evidence of this is found in the language used by social workers to describe the experiences of their clients. A study of a random selection of forms completed by social workers recording information about women referred to them for assessment under the Mental Health Act found few references to the circumstances of women's lives compared with references to medical diagnoses and 'failure to co-operate' with treatment (Barnes, Bowl and Fisher, 1990: 139).

Social work may in fact divert attention away from the mental health problems experienced by women who are also mothers by concentrating on child care problems. These are both more popular as a subject for intervention amongst social workers, and seen to be higher priority by social work managers. The legislative context of child care work is a reflection of society's view of the importance of such work and reinforces the priority given to it within social services departments. Fisher's *et al* study of mental health social work described clients' perceptions of social work input:

'There was, furthermore, very little in the clients' accounts of social work activity which could be construed as indicating an attempt to change those behaviour-patterns of clients which contributed to the degree of stress they experienced. For instance, one client described in detail her extensive contact with social workers as largely associated with her children's absence from school and their subsequent admission to care. She perceived the social worker as 'coming for the children' and not for her; she had come to understand that listening to her personal problems (which included agoraphobia and consequent isolation at home, relieved by the presence at home of her children) was 'not really part of the job'. (Fisher, Newton and Sainsbury, 1984: 113.)

Social work emphasis on child care may not always be neutral in its effect on mothers experiencing mental health problems. It may serve to define or underline her failure to be 'a good mother'. This in turn may increase the feelings of depression or worthlessness which are part of her problem. Simply by indicating that it is not part of the job is likely to reinforce her feeling that it is wrong to assert her own needs rather than those of the rest of the family. This and the often repeated finding that social workers are simply not good at noticing mental health difficulties in those referred to them (e.g. Cohen and Fisher, 1987) means that women do not generally, of choice, turn to a social worker for help with their mental distress.

One of us has described elsewhere (Maple, 1988) an attempt to concentrate social work input on a short term therapeutic intervention which specifically addresses mental health problems of social work clients. Amongst the clients involved were women whose 'cases' were defined as 'family/child care' cases and who were receiving little help directed solely at their personal problems rather than the child care problems. In one instance there had been considerable social work involvement over a number of years:

'Mrs D's case, for example, had been held by a long term worker for over eight years with much activity concentrated on statutory child care commitment focused on protecting the child's welfare. Whilst this has indeed provided a protection to safeguard the child's health and general welfare, it had also supported the child in an environment which had certainly contributed to Mrs D's own emotional problems (op.cit. p.23).

The findings of this small scale project suggest that if a commitment is made to addressing directly the mental health problems of the women involved this cannot only have advantages for the women themselves, but can also improve their ability to retain the care of their children. The need for long term social work intervention can thus be obviated. A major problem, however, is that current working practices as well as priorities do not lend themselves to the type of work required. We will return to a consideration of the organisational issues raised by this in the final chapter of this book.

Social work and other disciplines in the mental health field have been strongly influenced by psychoanalytic concepts both in the understanding of emotional distress and as a method of treatment. Fisher's *et al* study of two social work area teams (1984) supported this view. Despite innovations in practice in the 1970s when groupwork and community work were developed as alternative methods of social work intervention, the social work methods used by the workers in the study were almost exclusively traditional social casework oriented methods. Efforts aimed towards more social engineering remained very much on the periphery of the organisational ethos if they existed at all.

The resurgent feminist movement of the 1960s rejected the traditional psychoanalytic thinking on which social casework is based. Objections were made both to the tacit acceptance of male development as the norm in psychoanalysis as well as to the perceived difference in power positions between professional and client. The movement at that time believed that psychoanalysis aimed at the achievement of a better adjustment to traditional societal demands, the patriarchal values of which were identified with by the worker, who in turn would influence the client accordingly.

Certainly, much of the early psychoanalytic thinking was developed by men brought up in nineteenth-century European families where women's roles were strictly prescribed. Freud's difficult patient Dora, whom he found tantalising for her rejection of a male friend of her father and then himself, was a woman who did not behave in accordance with the female gender role stereotypes of the time nor did she assume the compliant patient role. His ideas of penis envy, of the castration complex in women, based on his sense of female sexuality as being the 'wrong' side of a coveted male sexualism, was pursued with sexist confidence:

> 'She acknowledges the fact of her castration, and with it too, the superiority of the male and her own inferiority; but she rebels against this unwelcome state of affairs . . . To an incredibly late age she clings to the hope of getting a penis some time.' (Freud, 1977: 376.)

Although he modified his views to some extent in later work, male envy of the breast, of femininity, of maternalism was not explored at all by this male thinker who has been so influential in our thinking about human development.

A reappraisal of the early Freudian view by later psychoanalysts, object relations theorists such as Klein, Fairbairn, Winnicott and Kohut, emphasised the developing child's need for relatedness as opposed to the Freudian idea of the satisfaction of libidinal, erotogenic drives. Their work, and that of John Bowlby, the child psychiatrist, has, over the years, greatly influenced views about early child development and the importance of the parental role in this, and thus the services needed to support families.

Arguments have raged about the concept of maternal deprivation which Bowlby developed and later modified. His subsequent work on attachment theory and the need for the child to have a secure base from which to explore the world with confidence was based on careful empirical study of a large number of case histories and, as such, is an appealing base from which to attempt to develop service strategies. Feminists have pointed to the irony that generations of mothers have been told how to behave by, and have attempted to

co-operate with, predominantly male specialists whose only
genuine experience of the intricacies of the mother/infant
relationships comes inevitably from only one viewpoint — that of
their experience of being a helpless child. So we welcome the
contributions to the debate that are now coming from women who
have actually experienced the relationship from both sides and are
beginning to write about the conflicts involved from their even more
expert perspective! (e.g. Ernst, 1987: 68–116; Olivier, 1989; Price,
1988; Rich, 1977).

Conclusion

In this chapter we have outlined some of the evidence concerning
women's experiences of mental health problems and the responses
of professional helpers to this. We hope we have provided enough
evidence to convince men as well as women workers in the 'mental
health professions' that awareness of gender difference should play
a key role both in understanding and responding to the needs of the
women referred to them and that such a response should neither be
gender blind nor based on assumptions about the appropriate role
and behaviour of the women concerned.

Drawing on the evidence we have presented in this chapter, we
feel there are a number of conditions necessary to the achievement
of a non-sexist mental health practice. These are: a willingness to
recognise stereotypical models of behaviour in ourselves and others,
a commitment to asking questions, and the will to learn from such
an informed analysis in order to make improvements in both current
and future services. Essentially, this has implications for the theory
base of practice, the personal, professional and practical issues
which derive from these as well as for the organisational
environment in which the work takes place.

We do not suggest that only women themselves can develop and
provide a good enough service truly to promote the interests of
women clients. Nor do we imply that there is only one answer. What
is clear, however, is that the development of a non-sexist practice
requires women's empowerment both as workers and clients and
these conditions may be more comfortably obtained in single gender
environments initially. In our view, there are long-lasting benefits

to be gained from a clear commitment to advance a theory and practice of gender egalitarian mental health practice which should ideally be provided by both men and women working within a variety of disciplines and settings.

If a genuinely non-sexist mental health practice is to be developed, the change for all involved is to work towards a position where the models of what is easier and most familiar for the worker can also contain the new understandings. To achieve this we must confront and challenge traditional mental health practice based on medical stereotypes, on unmodified psychoanalytic understandings and provided from an organisational base where sexist working relationships operate. We can then consider more effective modes of working wherever women's mental health needs are addressed. In this way, there is the opportunity now to further promote the mental health of both women users and women workers in the mental health system.

The Case Studies

In the following sections we use case studies of women known to us or the workers we have met in the course of our research for this book. Identifying details have been changed in order to protect their confidentiality.

The examples are of women experiencing emotional distress at various stages in their lives and who have come to the attention of social work or other mental health agencies. It is our belief that societal expectations of women at different ages and stages make particular demands for internal adjustments at such times. We believe that the present-day understanding of emotional distress and the social and psychological processes that affect this is still far from complete. So we attempt here to describe rather than use labels which can be misinterpreted and also contribute to discrimination.

Thus we begin with a description of the problems of the women we cite in our case examples which are common to many of those who are diagnosed as mentally disordered. We will then develop the relevant mental health issues together with a description of symptoms. We discuss symptoms in the context of our belief that being in touch with both comfortable and uncomfortable feelings, with sometimes uncontrollable emotions, is all part of a continuum of response to the experience of life and is a prerequisite for the maintenance of the mental health of all of us.

Alternative practices and models of intervention which challenge the stereotyping will be proposed based on our view that an effective non-sexist service for women with mental health problems will include a range of psychodynamic, social and medical responses. Such responses will be provided by a range of workers, from volunteers in self help groups, counsellors and therapists in voluntary and statutory agencies, to doctors and social workers working in the National Health Service and local authority departments. In the appendix we suggest questions which workers may wish to ask of themselves, their clients and their agencies, if they are to develop their practice in the direction we are proposing.

2. CHILDHOOD AND ADOLESCENCE: 'SEEN BUT NOT HEARD'

'Mine is a girl, but I don't really mind because you can dress 'em pretty' (Quoted by Vivienne Welburn in her book on post-natal depression, Welburn, 1980)

Good little girl

Although in Britain, in the 1990s, we congratulate the new parents warmly whether the child is male or female, many women carry with them the parental disappointment their gender can still evoke. The effect their 'second choice' quality can have on girl children and on the women they become, can be extremely damaging. In this chapter we will start to explore some of these impacts and their relevance for future mental health, focusing particularly on the effect of child physical and sexual abuse. We will also consider potentially less explicit forms of oppression which can lead to responses such as self-starvation or gorging of food.

The emphasis in our patriarchal society for female children to consider the needs of others and the family unit as a whole, at the expense of their own interests, leads to girl children being at the bottom of the pecking order in terms of power within many a family environment. In an illuminating diary (Grabucker, 1988) a feminist mother describes her attempt to raise her daughter differently from her own experience of upbringing.

'I did not want her to be compliant, to keep her opinions to herself and to smile sweetly instead of contradicting. I did not want her to be always checking and rethinking her ideas before daring to open her mouth, unlike her male counterparts who would say everything three times and then repeat it once again. And I did not want her to be completely devoted to some man who would be contin-ually finding fault with and criticising her until she lost faith in herself. I wanted her to avoid having plans for the future which were modest and which fitted in neatly with the reality of women's lives. My daughter was going to reach for the stars!'

So begins a revealing experience which describes how Grabucker's daughter learns which is the powerful gender in the world she has been born into. Grabucker describes how her daughter is shown that men are permitted to ignore people, to throw their weight around (just like a man, says the proud mother of a 2-year-old boy who is throwing sand in the playgroup) and how the skill and dexterity that girls demonstrate can be taken advantage of to get things done quickly until it is finally just taken for granted. The encouragement boys receive to explore their aggression is generally missing for girls. Similarly the girl child sees around her stereotypically submissive role models for her interaction both as a child and as an adult, yet she must still learn to deal with her own drives for personal power and autonomy.

No wonder Grabucker's little girl tries to become a boy. Even in her world, where she has a feminist minded mother, the male roles she sees around her are active, powerful and enviable by contrast to those of the female. '"In the eyes of the child the father embodies. . . . strength, the ideal, the outside world," said Winnicott (the psychoanalyst) generations ago. The mother is stuck in her daily routine, she embodies house and household. And women encourage this fantasy!' Grabucker suggests (Grabucker, 1988: 50), describing a holiday trip where anything out of the ordinary was put off until later with the comment, 'Daddy will do that with you' (op.cit.). Additionally, despite the work of Rutter and colleagues in dispelling the myth of the child being affected by mother's absence at work, many working mothers attempting to expand their roles still carry some guilt associated with this as well as the burden of the majority of household tasks (Rutter, 1971).

Clearly, an enormous amount can be done for the female child in the first few years, by the process of moulding, by domination, the teaching of acceptable habits and the punishment of perceived bad habits. Patterns of behaviour developed in childhood can have a powerful impact on adult relationships. Early experiences impact on emotional and behavioural disorder during childhood and contribute longer term to the mental health of the grown woman. For example, children and young people can feel a strong sense of responsibility for events over which they have no control and can experience considerable anxiety as a result. If a girl does not express her frustrations with dual standards in the care she receives in an overtly rebellious way, the result can be the internalisation of contradictions as evidence that it is her fault. The most saddening of all examples of this can be seen in the responses of some young girls who have been physically or sexually abused by trusted adults - often their fathers. Many abused women are unconsciously driven to recreate in their future families the painful but known ways of relating they learnt as a child.

Molly

Molly, the second youngest of a family of five children, had a father who was very ill with a heart condition for much of her childhood. She remembers him as dominating the family completely and describes coming home from school and having to read the paper to him instead of being allowed out to play. Her mother was very cowed as were the other children. Molly was the only one who dared to 'tell him the truth' and she was beaten for her pains. When he was dying, he told her he had 'only done it because I love you'. Ten years later, in her early 20s, Molly by now the mother of three children of her own, has spent the last six years trying to separate from a husband who was not only physically violent on several occasions but has also raped her twice in front of the children. He tells her 'I only do this because I love you and you love me'. Unknowingly, Molly was repeating in adulthood the pattern of family relationships she had learnt as a child.

Molly felt that no one wanted to know about her pain, either then or now. She reported both the rape experiences to the police but when she first went to court her husband was very patronising and the judge equally so, dismissing the case and calling her a 'silly, hysterical woman'. In the second incident, the Crown Prosecution Service decided there was insufficient evidence to pursue the matter.

Fortunately, a recent court case, which has set a precedent within the British legal system, where a man was convicted and sentenced for raping his wife whilst they were still married, may hold out some hope for women such as Molly. But there is clearly a long way to go before women's voices are properly heard.

If the female child is allowed to react appropriately when she is distressed or in pain, whether physical or psychological, then she has the chance of overcoming the serious consequences of early experiences. If the adults around the child, however, cannot tolerate the expression of anger, sadness or distress and teach repression or the child to collude guiltily, neurotic symptoms may develop. The psychoanalyst Alice Miller, in her book entitled For Your Own Good, graphically describes the suffering inflicted on children under the heading of Child Rearing (Miller, 1987). She identifies the resulting conflict in the young child who, experiencing harsh treatment from the caretaker on whom she is completely dependent for survival, internalises and denies her feelings beneath the over riding need to believe in the caretaker's inherent goodness. Fairbairn, one of the pioneers of object relations theory, suggests eloquently that, for the small, scared child it perhaps seems more bearable to think of herself as a bad person in a world ruled by God, than as a good person in a world ruled by the devil! (Fairbairn, in Buckley, 1986: 102—126)

The story of Christiane F. is an example of this. Christiane's father beat her regularly for reasons she did not understand but which she later came to explain derived from his feeling of failure in business. She finally becomes addicted to drugs and thus provides a good reason for the beatings she has already received.

> 'This is the only way she has to rescue the image of a father she loves and idealizes. She also begins to provoke other men and turn them into punitive fathers — first the building superintendent, then her teachers and finally, during her drug addiction, the police. In this way she can shift the conflict with her father onto other people.' (Miller 1987: 112–113.)

Miller studied child-rearing practices in general and identified the suffering of both male and female children caused by parents asserting their powerful status in respect of their children. Information gathered in 1989 suggests that 85% of British parents regularly beat their children (Jowell, Witherspoon and Brook).

Miller (1984) proposes that, because we all have the experience of the powerlessness of a child and still perhaps unconsciously wish 'to get our own back', we choose to remain unaware of the consequences of this practice for us all. Society's wishes to remain 'unaware' have been demonstrated graphically by the painful experiences of all involved in the recent controversies related to child sexual abuse in Cleveland and elsewhere. The workers involved in attempting to help children suspected of being sexually abused were themselves subjected to public condemnation and abuse far greater than their mistakes deserved. (Campbell, 1988.)

Child physical abuse and particularly child sexual abuse is predominantly an act of male domination over female children within the home. Disclosure of abuse can lead to female children being made to feel guilty and responsible for family breakdown. One of us came across a woman in her 40s who had been in and out of psychiatric hospitals all her adult life. Her notes described something of her history; one of a large family, at the age of nine she had been sexually abused by her brother. She had reported the abuse and as a result her brother was convicted and sent to prison. Whilst in prison he had died in dubious circumstances. She had subsequently been rejected by the rest of the family as being responsible for the death of a favourite son.

Because of such pressures, it is often only when a child leaves the family for other reasons that the knowledge of the abuse becomes accessible and transmittable to others.

Marie

Marie was the oldest daughter of a family of five children living in a large council house with their mother, grandmother and stepfather and various pets. The family were well known to the helping agencies in the area who were concerned about the physical conditions in the home and some acting out behaviour on the part of the older children. Apart from appalling hygiene, the whole family seemed warm, loving and caring of each other, with Marie's stepfather managing to hold down a responsible job and to keep up a reasonable appearance despite all the odds apparently being against him. Initial social work intervention was marital work aimed at improving the marriage. This met with some apparent success and Mr. M., the stepfather assumed a greater responsibility for the day-to-day affairs in the home. The workers involved saw him as the most approachable, stable and insightful member of the family and their work was clearly directed towards helping him maintain his position there.

Subsequent to the marital intervention, the social worker, in conjunction with the other health and education workers involved with the family, attempted a close supervision aimed at improving the self image of the family as a whole, and Marie's mother in particular, Mrs. M., suffered from depression and gynaecological problems and this was considered contributory to her inability to motivate herself to do more to care for her family. Tranquillisers were prescribed by the GP and a subsequent hysterectomy took place. Intensive cleaning up in the home was followed by regular sessions aimed at helping the family develop and maintain a reasonable domestic routine. When this failed and the children were again being ostracised at school because of their appearance and smell, the local authority decided to initiate care proceedings. Overnight, the family tidied up and Mr. M. redecorated, new clean clothes were bought for all the children and the family promised to improve their standards. The request for a court hearing was withdrawn in consequence. Marie's mother, who was always happier out of the house, found a part-time job and Marie at 14 found a boy friend who was encouraged by Mrs. M. to become 'part of the family'. The local authority resumed a monitoring role and, guided by the wish to keep the family together because of the emotional support it was felt this provided for its members, minimal standards of child care were tolerated. It was not until Marie at 16 was in hospital having her first baby that she told the social worker that Mr. M. had been abusing her sexually for years.

Marie's story remains a sad one. The paternity of the baby was never successfully established and she has not been able successfully to bond with him. Currently, he is being placed for adoption. Marie herself has not as yet been able to share much of her feelings about her experiences and still views the professional workers as unhelpful and probably hostile. Here, stereotyping had played a considerable part in maintaining an 'abuse' situation. Mr. M. was relatively hardworking, amenable and clearly fond of the children. His presence in the house was considered a very positive factor by the workers who identified Mrs. M. as the difficult partner. She certainly did not live up to her stereotypical caring role. Much effort was aimed at helping her to do so whilst the chaos in the home itself illustrated Mrs. M.'s feelings about herself as well as providing a diversion and a smokescreen which kept the workers at arm's length from the abuse.

If we as child care workers, mental health workers, teachers, neighbours and the public generally are to combat child abuse we must learn to listen to children. We must ignore the cultural pre-conditioning that tempts us to remain unaware. If Marie's social worker had acted on her hunch to spend more time with Marie on her own as well as recognising her own stereotyping behaviour, she might well have been able to offer her greater protection much earlier. As the prevalence of child abuse, whether in physical, sexual or even ritualised forms, is becoming increasingly recognised, child care agencies are recognising the need for increased specialist training for staff in the sensitive areas of early recognition and disclosure work.

Margaret Jervis (1991), in an article written three years after the judicial inquiry into the Cleveland crisis, identified some of the contextual issues which remain unacknowledged and unaddressed. In the Cleveland area, unemployment remains two and a half times the national average. Serial monogamy and reconstituted families are an emerging form of normality in an area which has always considered itself a 'rough and tough place' and where the masculine ethos has remained dominant throughout the years of boom and recession. Jervis suggests the 'war of the sexes meanders through the story of the Cleveland crisis', with a 'lot of latent support for the professionals among the women, whilst men still tend to be defensive about the whole issue.' (p14)

She concludes:

> 'What would have been the focus (of public concern) if most of the families affected in Cleveland had been black? My guess is that acres of print would have been expended on the cultural context, the lack of sensitivity, the absence of knowledge. Transpose black for white disinherited

working class and little or no attention is paid. We assume
we know. Perhaps its time we started finding out' (p.15).

No amount of increased sensitivity training, child care
procedures or child abuse registers will protect our children unless
there is also a willingness to recognise our own prejudices and
stereotyping and to work towards a society where oppression and
abuse are acknowledged as belonging to us all. Removing children
from one abusing home to another setting where poorly trained and
undervalued residential staff or foster parents are left without
adequate support to deal with a number of traumatised children may
be abuse of another kind. Preventing both further abuse and the
repetition of abusing behaviour in future relationships requires a
commitment to working with the child therapeutically. She will
need help to understand what has happened and her part within it
in order to experience appropriate responses and then move beyond
them. If it is possible to communicate with victims when the
experience is fresh, we can help to prevent some of the future
relationship difficulties abused women describe.

Workers in the mental health field are increasingly identifying
the impact that abuse as a child, and sexual abuse in particular, can
have on the future mental health of the victims. One worker we
spoke to whilst gathering material for this book suggested that 85%
of her adult women counselling clients had suffered some form of
abuse. And although it is still difficult to be certain of the reality
of the extent of abuse of children, in an as yet unpublished study
Tyrell Harris reported more figures to a recent conference on the
'Effect of Relationships on Relationships'. She had found that out
of 147 women psychiatric patients she interviewed, 54 had suffered
sexual abuse as children.

Briere suggests that the long term emotional difficulties
experienced following childhood abuse can be similar to those of
the psychiatric diagnosis 'borderline personality disorder'. This is
a diagnosis that still arouses debate but currently can be taken to
mean someone whose symptoms and behaviour are not easily
categorised but can seem to be on the borderline between neurosis
(this term covers conditions such as anxiety and depression) and
psychosis (this term covers conditions such as schizophrenia and
paranoia). The difference between these two major terms of

psychiatric classification is related to how much understanding of the reality of their situation the sufferer has. The criteria for the borderline personality disorder diagnosis involve a cluster of symptoms such as anxiety attacks, sleep disturbances and nightmares, feelings of isolation, problems with anger, parasuicidal and self-mutilatory behaviour, drug abuse, alcoholism. A failure to develop basic trust in those around them, a sense of exploitation and violation and a poor self image related to feelings of guilt and shame experienced by survivors of abuse are all consistent with this picture. Alice's story, for example, is one where her carers, both family and professional, have let her down.

Alice

Alice, now 35 years old, has been in a long term ward in a psychiatric hospital since she was 16, following an admission subsequent to an attempted suicide. Her parents, both alive at the time of admission, are now dead and her brother suffers from schizophrenia. Her current diagnosis is 'burnt out schizophrenic' and she presents with the common medication side effects of involuntary movement and mannerisms. The ward staff describe her as self-abusive and she can be violent to others. She often attempts to deny her femininity, refusing to admit that she has periods and even that she is a woman. She is considered promiscuous and vulnerable to exploitation.

Many long term patients have been re-evaluated in the current climate of closure of the large institutions and the move towards community care. A recent examination of Alice's notes by a staff member appointed to this task identified these details from Alice's experiences:

> 'She claimed to have been sexually abused by her father, brother and a lodger. When she was first admitted, nurses reported that her father was seen adjusting his clothes after visiting her and she was found to have her skirt up.
>
> The male consultant psychiatrist felt sexual abuse was "not the sort of thing that happened in that sort of (apparently strongly religious) family".'

The notes stated that after the children were born Alice's mother was no longer interested in sex and Alice's father felt at times that he was a 'nuisance to his wife'.

At the ward round, the main interest in Alice was (and remains) how she ate and slept and responded to her medication, 'anything strange' in terms of Alice's ₌nments was (and still is) responded to as 'the illness speaking' and her medication would be changed.

For Alice it may well be too late. Her story was not heard by those who might have been in a position to help at the time and 15 years later she is seen as too ill to manage or be managed in the community. For others, there may be more chance if the professionals can bear to hear.

For a successful therapeutic response, workers must be prepared to face a considerable challenge from such women who have been so misused by trusted carers in the past. Particular implications for the social work relationship will be particularly centred upon the woman's strong unmet dependency needs, her testing of the relationship boundaries and a desire for personal contact with the worker. A successful working relationship would, we believe, need to contain the following elements: the achievement and maintenance of empathy, an experience of being held and validated whilst being offered non-intrusive, empowering caring. These qualities within the worker's intervention should allow eventually for some positive reparatory work to be done.

One attempt to put these principles into practice has been made in an initiative which involved both the local social services area team and a voluntary agency, the Family Services Unit. A group for sexually abused young women, aged 13 to 17, was led by a social worker from each setting. The group aimed to create an atmosphere of safety and trust for the young women where they could explore their feelings about their experiences as well as express their anger and confusion about those who should have cared for them and who had betrayed their trust. It was hoped that this would help to improve their self-confidence and at the same time decrease the feelings of isolation experienced by many abuse survivors.

The pilot stage of this group ran for 12 weekly sessions and had an average membership of five young women. Much negotiation was involved in the establishment of the group in terms of accountability issues and support for the group leaders. A planned programme for the group included exercises, activities, games and role play as well as the exploration of group processes.

All members were interviewed by the group leaders prior to commencement. In the course of the pilot group members spoke of their feelings about not being believed, about the process of the investigations into the abuse and about the legal system. Relationships in their families were explored and important issues such as trust and mistrust, power and authority were raised and developed. As safety and trust in the group itself developed, the young women were also able to explore issues around their own sexuality and to acknowledge appropriately for the first time, the anger they felt. For some this anger had been turned in on themselves in the form of self-harm. At the end of the programme of group sessions, the group members spoke of the impact the group had had for them:

> 'Before I came to the group I could not speak about me being sexually abused to anyone, not even my parents.'

> 'I have been able to talk to my parents about me being sexually abused as where before I couldn't . . .It also makes me realise that I am not the only person who has been abused as I thought I was, and that is why I didn't tell anyone until some while later about me being abused.'

> 'I can now walk down the street without feeling that everybody is looking at me and knows that I have been sexually abused.'(Gray and Swindell, 1987.)

Feedback from one of the social workers with case responsibility for a group member was as follows: 'It is abundantly clear in P's case that the group has provided the stimulus for change and progress that has been lacking through structured contact with psychologists/social workers over several years.'

The group experience described here involved liaison between two agencies, with shared responsibility for management. Joint meetings were held throughout the project, and time was made available for the workers to plan their joint work and to evaluate progress. Premises were made available by the voluntary organisation but transport of group members to the project and home again was provided by the social services department. It was a particularly stressful piece of work for the workers concerned as the topic inevitably raised their own feelings about the abuse of power and authority and the group members brought with them patterns of relating to carers that were conflictual and divisive. For this reason access to a groupwork consultant for support was essential.

Swindell (forthcoming) identifies the following features as contributory to the effectiveness of the model of intervention used:

1. Humanistic values such as client empowerment through participation in contracting and evaluation.

2. Psychodynamic theory as a framework for understanding what is happening.

3. Groupwork as a method which counteracts isolation and harnesses peer group influences.

4. Clear accountability contracts.

5. The provision of alternative experiences, in particular, protection, clear boundaries, open communication, empowerment, trust, respect for the individual and age appropriate responsibility.

6. The opportunity for awareness and expression of repressed feelings, which is essential for therapeutic healing.

7. Relationship of trust built up between group leaders and members over a period of time.

8. Planning, feedback and consultancy structures for co-working.

9. Awareness of effect on workers and provision of support. (p.14.)

The group provided a creative, preventive response to abused young women in a way that had very positive ramifications for their future mental health and further groups were established on the lines of this pilot project. The cost of the service was greater than a traditional social work service would have been. We are convinced, however, that the increased investment at this early stage is justifiable, not only in terms of the the avoidance of long term mental distress for the young women themselves, but also as a way of avoiding the possible repetition of abusing behaviour in future generations.

Slag or slut?

A young girl growing up in a world in which male definitions of correct behaviour predominate has some hard lessons to learn. This is often particularly acute during adolescence when awareness of gender relations and of sexuality starts to influence attitudes towards many aspects of life (see Lees, 1989). Girls can become increasingly conscious of the bases on which their behaviour is being judged. That such judgements are often unfair is acknowledged but few can resist their force.

The way a girl dresses as well as the number of boyfriends she has can lead to the application of one of a large number of derogatory terms which do not have real equivalents in terms applied to boys. The fear of being labelled in this way is a strong form of social control and the only way out, it seems, is to 'go steady' with one boy. Her behaviour is then subject to the control of one particular male as well as to more-generalised social controls. Her opportunity to explore her emerging individuality and sexuality is not tolerated in the way that it is amongst her male contemporaries and any expression of deviance in this respect is likely to receive a more repressive response, ostensibly for her own protection.

Sue Lees studied the views of 15-and 16-year-olds about school, friendship, marriage and the future. Although aware from their mothers' experiences that 'marriage was something you ended up with after you had lived', these girls saw little option in their lives other than to marry in order to obtain a valued position in the world.

41

The period in which adolescent girls are becoming aware of and trying to make sense of their future options as women can be difficult not only because of the need to come to terms with new feelings and experiences that are happening now, but also because of an awareness that they have only a short space in which they can 'be themselves' before they have to become what is expected of them. The response to that can be varied:

> 'There is evidence in these pages that some girls, some-
> times, become aware of a discrepancy between the dis-
> course and themselves, between who they are told they
> are and who, in some inchoate way (because lacking a
> conventional language of expression), they feel them-
> selves to be — at least as a for ever possibility, closed off
> but whimsically and fleetingly grasped. This may pro-
> duce insanity . . . . A few of the permanently marginalised
> remain angry . . . . But most of the girls we write about
> resolve the contradiction by resignation and compliance.'
> (Cain 1989: 5.)

Adolescence is a time when a cry for help can take many forms. Some young women collude with society's image of an acceptable female body shape by restricting their food intake. Others reject parental and social values in a more overt way. We consider both such responses below. But underlying any 'deviant' behaviour is the need for all young women successfully to make the transition to independence. To do this, it seems there is a need to resolve some of their ambivalence about dependence on their family of origin and the values to which this family ascribe. If we believe in the 'self-in-relation' model for womens development, Hartman (1989) suggests that we should help young women at this stage to aim for 'leaving home without leaving home'. In other words, we need to look for models of independence within relationships which aim to encourage women to develop their own identities in a creative way whilst maintaining mature interdependent relationships with others. The mood swings of adolescence, which can veer rapidly from the deepest depression to the heights of euphoria, from love to hate, as the young adult explores and compares her family and the world in which she is about to take a full place, can be difficult to

42

understand and tolerate. Parents may well have their own concerns at this time — the mid-time of their lives coinciding with the beginning of the adulthood of their daughter (see p.74). A high percentage of diagnosed schizophrenic breakdowns occur in adolescence and we believe this must be linked to the developmental stage, both to physical changes and to the dilemmas of trying to relate to changing individual perceptions of self and family with an increasing awareness of societal expectations.

Adolescent girls whose deviance is defined as delinquency can expect to receive different treatment within the criminal justice system from their male peers (see, for example, Hudson, A. 1988, Hudson, B, 1989 and Gelsthorpe, 1985). This mirrors the situation in the mental health system. Criminal behaviour amongst boys and young men is considered 'normal', whereas the same behaviour in girls is considered 'abnormal' and as evidence of some deep-seated psycho-social problem.

Hence the judgements made of a young woman who offends can be very similar to the judgements made of those experiencing mental health problems and the response in both cases can be designed to reassert normal feminine characteristics and the fulfilment of the appropriate female role.

'Troublesome' girls can cause great problems for welfare professionals. Outbursts of aggression and sullen containment of discontent can be regarded as indications of deficiencies in their personalities rather than expressions of their awareness of the injustices they are experiencing. The project manager of a specialist service provided for girls and young women by a local authority social services department suggested that part of the reason for this relates to the difficulty experienced by women in getting themselves and their concerns appropriately heard. The vast majority of the clients of this service come from single parent families where the parents seem like adolescents themselves. Young women come to the project saying, 'We want you to listen'. Daughters can be seen as competition by their mothers. Sexuality can be a very big issue in families where the mothers themselves are without partners and are jealous of their daughters. The fact that *their* mothers had also never been listened to tends to compound the problem as they struggle to persuade teachers and police to appreciate the difficulties with their daughters. In those families where there are two partners, stereotypical role expectations mean Dad is the parent who is usually out but who makes the decisions. Mum takes the responsibility for child care and is blamed when the daughter acts out.

The project mentioned above, the Maya Project supported by the London Borough of Hammersmith, aims to assist young women to develop in self-confidence and assertiveness, to provide positive images of womanhood, challenge discrimination and provide support to young women in families at risk of breakdown. It does this through various activities - keyworking with individual young women, group and family work, counselling and groupwork with sexually abused young women, training and consultancy to other workers. One of their most successful ventures is a group entitled 'What she wants'. Here young women are encouraged to identify their needs, both in their families and the outside world, and to work on appropriate strategies for achieving their aims. Much of the focus is on how to deal more successfully with their own and other people's anger, an understandable need for young women growing up in a society where they feel oppressed on all counts. It is also an opportunity for young women to relate in a setting without the competitive element that can exist for them in the outside environment. Young women rarely have the support that young men can have from single gender 'gangs'. They are not encouraged to hang about in groups nor generally choose to because of the ethos of 'you must get a man' which can set up competition and separates the individual from her peers.

This project also provides specific groups for young women from ethnic minorities and lesbians, both of which are seen to have special needs to gain support from others in similar circumstances and to explore, in a confidential setting, issues which might elsewhere seem taboo, for example, black women's views of black men.

Eating Disorders

Eating disorders appear to have become more prevalent in recent years, although, as with child abuse, the possibility is that the phenomenon has been with us for many years without being properly recognised. Lawrence and Dana (1990), for example, acknowledge that whilst the incidence of eating disorders has increased dramatically in the past 20 years and may well be connected to the particular social demands made upon women during this time, our understanding of the origins of the syndrome may be assisted by evidence from the Victorian era. In the 1870s, a time when it was believed that women's physical and mental constitution made them unsuitable for any kind of physical or intellectual activity, middle class women in large numbers began to suffer from a series of symptoms including fainting, weakness and loss of appetite.

Whilst opportunities for women may well have improved in the past two decades, the societal preference for women to seem powerless and childlike remains a powerful cultural pressure upon girls searching for an adult female role with which to feel comfortable. Jenny, the 15-year-old, whose story we tell below, had two ideal role models: Madonna and Marilyn Monroe. Both of these women seem to epitomise elements of an abused victim, child/woman persona. Stereotypical images of successful women in our society are rarely attractive and positive. The idealised body image for the adult woman in our Western culture can also only be attained by the average mature female by putting considerable restraints on her freedom. A recent study found that 75% of a group of 161 schoolgirls between the ages of 12 and 18 already restricted what they ate in an attempt to control their weight (Parry-Crooke and Ryan, 1986).

Jenny

Jenny was 15 and underweight when she was referred to a therapist by her local general practitioner. In her family, her grandfather, father and 2-years-older brother Robert, all suffered from severe life-threatening illnesses when Jenny was young. Father and brother were asthmatic and Jenny remembers lying in bed at night, hearing her brother struggling for breath and, frightened he might die, hoping that someone would come to soothe her fears. Instead mother would be looking after Robert, or her husband or, when Jenny was 14, grandfather who came to die from emphysema. Jenny and Robert seem to have acted out the unhappiness in the family through their sibling rivalry throughout their short lives. Robert, who was very badly behaved at home, is now at boarding school. He is overweight and liable to dramatic outbursts. He was once found drunk at school and needed to be rushed to hospital. He somehow always seems able to enlist attention.

For most of the time, Jenny is quiet and good as if by contrast she keeps her feelings inside. Certainly she attempts to control her food intake and thus remain outwardly in control. Robert tells Jenny that she is fat and ugly and will never get a man. When he attacks her like this she wants to vomit, so when she is alone, she rushes to the cupboards, stuffs herself with crisps, biscuits, etc. and subsequently vomits. It took a visit from a family friend to bring Jenny's eating to her parents' attention.

Anorexia nervosa - literally 'a nervous loss of appetite' - can occur at any age, in any social class and there are a growing number of male sufferers. It is a serious condition characterised by a conflict between a frantic preoccupation with food and an active restraint from eating. Attendant features such as amenorrhea (loss of periods) may be related to the psychological condition or the result of extreme weight loss. Medical, surgical and obstetric complications are common and the children of women with anorexia nervosa are also at risk (Treasure, 1990). Many women do not respond well to present methods of treatment and deaths do occur. The majority of sufferers are girls and young women, many of whom are high achievers. Amongst them are many young women from families originating from the Asian sub-continent. The typical anorexia sufferer will be the girl described by her parents as hitherto compliant, passive and unselfish: 'She's never been any trouble until now'.

There is still much work to be done before we fully understand the causes of anorexia but Lawrence and Dana (1990) suggest that anorexic behaviour occurs in women who have developed a difficulty about tolerating and expressing the dependent, needy, childlike part of themselves. Thus the struggles of dependence versus autonomy and separation at adolescence may well be the trigger for the large number of anorexic girls of this age. Jenny's story above, the good, quiet daughter whose own neediness never seemed able to be properly acknowledged within the overburdened family, appears to bear this out. When investigated by the therapist, her description of bingeing on large amounts of food and then vomiting (symptoms of bulimia nervosa which can often be combined in anorexia sufferers), involved very small amounts of food, indicating that Jenny, like other young women with anorexia, had probably lost her sense of perspective about food and also her body size.

Sheila Macleod, who wrote about her own experience of anorexia nervosa over 20 years (Macleod, 1981), recognised that as a robust child with a younger sister who suffered from a weak chest, she 'learned the lesson even then that the frail receive more love and attention than the healthy'. What the sufferer herself usually does not recognise is that this struggle to gain freedom from her needy self and its yearnings, is in reality a serious psychological disorder which can have life-threatening consequences.

The other side of Jenny's response, overeating and then being sick, is unfortunately relatively common in women-overconcerned about their weight. This may become a way of life, with the woman eating and making herself sick as many as 15 times a day. The condition of bulimia, where the sufferer appears to have a normal weight and outward appearance, whilst secretly her life is out-of-control, may well represent the woman's inner conflicts. Part of her may appear to be outwardly competent and coping whilst the part of her that is full of fears and anxieties is well hidden and only surfaces in this out of control syndrome. Similarly, with compulsive eating, which too can be identified as a psychological problem of self-abuse often first recognised at adolescence, it is important to identify the fears and feelings that the food and the process of the disorder represent. In her book, Fat is a Feminist Issue, Susie Orbach proposes that 'fat is about protection, sex, nurturance, strength, boundaries, mothering, substance, assertion and rage' and sees compulsive eating as an attempt to respond to the conflicts women experience in their social environment (Orbach, 1978).

Many of the traditional responses to young women suffering from eating disorders have aimed at treating the symptoms rather than trying to understand and address the meanings behind these. Thus eating-disordered patients have been admitted to hospital and attempts have been made to institute disciplines related to either increasing or decreasing intake in various ways. Some of these methods, based on behavioural modification, have seemed almost as punishing as the self-abuse itself and relapses after such treatment are common. More recently, workers in various settings have attempted to listen to their patients and to understand the motivation behind the presenting symptoms whilst offering them the opportunity to explore the feelings their behaviour had attempted to repress.

What women with eating disorders have in common is their difficulty in ingesting food at an appropriate rate for their daily needs. Not surprisingly they experience similar problems with taking in and accepting therapeutic help, which equally can seem symbolically intrusive, insufficient or inappropriate. It is clear that the professional services have not yet established how best to respond to the increasing numbers of women who are referred to them suffering from eating disorders. The London Women's Therapy Centre, for example, is exploring various therapy settings, both individual and group, facilitated and self-help, and suggests that as far as is possible it is important that the woman herself should be able to choose what suits her best and that any intervention would need to be long term.

Jenny's therapist struggled to provide Jenny with a therapy programme that would allow them both to begin to know the needy child inside that had been unacknowledged for so long. At this stage, the therapist was aware of wanting to provide a perfect therapy experience for her young patient. Sharing her worries about this in her supervision group, enabled the worker to realise that she was tuning into Jenny's drive for perfection and she was then able to relax. The important experience for Jenny was to spend time with a therapist who could bear her needy feelings and provide a 'good enough' holding environment to allow for these to be explored.

Summary

Our patriarchal society treats its female children in oppressive ways which threaten their inherent self-confidence and basic trust. Girls and young women growing up within such a framework, where their needs are not heard or considered, may well respond to such pressures in ways that overtly demonstrate their sense of powerlessness, for example in a loss of, or an exaggeration of, emotional control. Traditionally, society has reinforced the view that this is unacceptable and has provided services that aim at restoring the discriminatory *status quo* whilst doing little to promote future mental health.

Our examples above are a few instances of those influences among many, which can have a considerable impact on the current and future mental health of any girl or young woman. Clearly the underlying message is the need for these young people to be heard and validated in their own right, and with their own rights. A non-sexist approach by workers involved, we believe, would include new ways of communicating both by worker and client such as Swindell describes, as well as addressing assertively the wider issues of female status both within the family and in the outside society.

3. ADULT WOMANHOOD/CHILDBEARING —
'Ideal Wife and Mother: Superwoman or Failure?'

'... the stereotype that women are passive is less a logical analysis than a wish fulfilment, which installs men in a dominant position. We might ask whether women have supported these stereotypes? And the answer surprisingly is yes, not simply because the culture conditions them to do so but because we are all, women and men, unconsciously overwhelmed by the omnipotent . . . mother, still trying to separate from her and afraid . . .'(Baruch & Sevanno 1988, 12).

Despite changing times, stereotypes of the traditional male and female roles are still successfully instilled into children from an early age and at all ages more girl children than boy children express a desire for children of their own (see Fransella and Frost, 1977). There are, in theory, more opportunities for women to work, certainly more expectations and often great financial pressure, which combine to encourage women to develop careers of some form. Paid employment also appears to provide some protection from the symptoms of depression (Cochrane and Stopes-Roe, 1981). Yet a major priority for most women in early adulthood remains the development of a stable relationship within which they can pursue the role of wife and mother. Although single women apparently experience less mental distress leading to hospital admission than do single men (Cochrane and Stopes-Roe, ibid), both the unmarried and the childless states still have more negative connotations for women than they do for men.

In her study of the transition to motherhood, Ann Oakley identified a thread of 'chronic self-doubt' running through interviews with the women concerned (Oakley, 1980). Coming from a basis of low self-esteem, women have a strong need for affiliation, and hope, as do men, that the love, approval and nurturance they seek can be achieved through partnership or marriage. They also hope and expect that motherhood will both confirm and enhance their status and identity as women.

The problem in both instances is that the reality, especially for women, is often at odds with the expectation.

It is significant that we know much less about the division of labour within households than we do about the changing position of women within the labour market. We have already noted that the way in which relationships between married couples are conducted and regulated is seen to be an essentially private matter. Not only has rape within marriage only recently become legally defined as possible, the police are also reluctant to intervene in cases of domestic violence. The British Social Attitudes report (Jowell, Witherspoon and Brook, 1988) provides depressing evidence for those wanting to believe that gender roles are undergoing real change. Both domestic and childcare tasks are still undertaken primarily by women: women had the main responsibility for preparing the evening meal in 77% of cases, for doing the household cleaning in 72%, doing the washing and ironing in 88% and for looking after sick children in 67% of cases.

The report does identify some shift in attitudes towards traditional roles in terms of women's rights to work outside the home. Even so, over one-fifth of respondents 'disagreed strongly' with the statement: 'Married women have a right to work if they want to, whatever their family situation.' And whilst a majority thought that it is better for a woman herself to have a job, only 14% agreed that this was better for the woman and her family. There has been a fundamental shift since 1965 in the attitude of women themselves towards their rights to paid employment. In 1965, 78% of women felt that mothers of children under five should not go out to work, whereas that had dropped to 45% in the most recent survey. However, such a change in attitudes has not been accompanied by an equivalent change in the availability of child care services to enable mothers to work and know that their children are receiving good quality care.

The benefits deriving from both the recognition and companionship that work outside the home can bring have to be balanced against the extra pressures. Whilst domestic tasks are more likely to be shared in those households where women work full-time outside the home, the situation for women who work part-time is similar to that for women who are not in paid employment. Extra responsibilities outside the home are not balanced by a lessening of responsibilities within it.

The Policy Studies Institute reported in 1990 that one in nine families struggle with debt and we know from the Social Attitudes survey that women are more likely than men to have responsibility for organising household money and bills. The stresses associated with administering an income which is insufficient to meet basic family needs are more often borne by women. One outcome of this is often a denial to herself, not only of 'luxuries' such as new clothes, but also necessities such as food. Becoming 'just a housewife' brings with it not only negative images . . . .

> 'She's one of them — with the rollers in her hair. Oh, I don't know what you're supposed to feel like when you are a housewife, I really don't . . . . But I know that housewife doesn't sound very interesting '(quoted in Oakley, 1980) . . . .

but also practical difficulties and a subordination of personal needs to those of partner and family.

A disjuncture between the expectations and reality of motherhood can provide an additional source of emotional stress during this period of women's lives. Fransella and Frost consider a variety of theories which have been put forward about the relationship between childbirth and emotional illness and suggest that there are many theories but little knowledge about why tension, depression and anxiety frequently attend pregnancy and childbirth. They do suggest that what might not have occurred to many theorists is that 'women might just be plain anxious about what is to happen to them' (Fransella and Frost, 1977: 161). They quote research which demonstrates that emotional problems were experienced more often by those having their second or third child than by those having their first, suggesting that women had learnt from experience that childbirth and motherhood are not unequivocally positive experiences.

Nor can women rely on sensitivity to their needs from the professionals who care for them at this stage. Hoppe (1985: 131) quotes from a selection of gynaecology textbooks published in the period from 1943 to 1972:

'The fundamental urge of women is motherhood balanced by the fact that sexual pleasure is entirely secondary or absent.'

'If there had been too much masturbation of the clitoris it may be reluctant to abandon control, or the vagina may be unwilling to accept the combined role of arbiter of sensation and vehicle for reproduction.'

'An important feature of sex desire in the man is the urge to dominate the woman and subjugate her to his will. In a woman, acquiescence to the masterful takes high place.'

At the very least these statements, which have influenced doctors still practising, reflect a serious lack of knowledge about their women patients. They also suggest attitudes that make it very unlikely that women will receive optimal, understanding health care at a very important time for them.

Ann Oakley's study of women making the 'Transition to Motherhood' provides a convincing discussion and explanation of what this experience really means to women (Oakley 1980). She considers childbirth as a life event which involves loss as well as gain and which requires the construction of new meanings if the gains are to outweigh the losses. Specifically the loss to a woman is an erosion of her personal identity. The way she is treated and seen by others is mediated by her role as a mother and for 69% of the women in this study their treatment as a mother was less favourable than their treatment as individual women.

At the same time, the physical exhaustion of early childcare and the emotional work required to deal with three way relationships rather than the one to one couple relationship represent additional pressures. Five months after the birth of their child, 47% of the women reported that the emotional closeness of their relationship with their partner had decreased, 42% said that satisfaction with masculine participation in housework had decreased and 51% that their satisfaction with masculine participation in childcare had decreased.

Contrasting the reality of the experience with a rosy view of the satisfactions of motherhood can make it all the more difficult. One response can be to hold oneself responsible for being stupid enough to believe the image. Another is to blame other women, midwives, childbirth educators and all those who have conspired to present an inaccurate and incomplete picture both of the experience of pregnancy and childbirth and of motherhood itself.

Oakley (who has three children herself) suggests that the only reason women do not break down completely after childbirth is that the outcome of their labour is the love, development and growth of another human being. This in itself can contribute to rather than detract from self-esteem, although it is not inevitable nor immediate. She concludes:

> 'Life events constitute loss events if their major effect is to deprive a person of sources of value or reward. Faced with such deprivation, a person may struggle on and emerge without disabling emotional impairment if he/she feels in control of the parameters of his/her life space and is able to exercise this control effectively, so as to restore a sense of meaning. Otherwise the response to loss is liable to be hopelessness and the risk of feeling this way for very long is its generalisation; in such generalisation of hopelessness probably lies the genesis of clinical depression (and other states thus labelled by their possessors).' (Oakley, 1980: 251.)

Griefwork to respond to the sense of their lost identity may therefore be as necessary for mothers at this time of their lives as following bereavement. It is certainly clear that the years of young adult womanhood and childbearing are not an easy stage in any woman's life. For some women 'post-natal depression' or 'puerperal psychosis' (in the medical jargon) can be the result. In other cases unresolved conflicts at this stage can lead to difficulties later on. The adjustments required by parenthood may also be difficult for fathers and this can in itself create additional needs for adjustment within the relationship. Social workers working with women experiencing mental distress as a result of the adjustments required by motherhood may find themselves involved in helping them make sense of changed relationships with their partners as well.

Adjusting to Parenthood

Ray and Jackie

Ray was 38 years old, married with two children, a girl aged 8 and a boy aged 18 months, when he was first referred for social work support. He told the worker the story of his recent experiences. Just at the time that his baby son was born he became unemployed. Up until then he had worked long hours on night shift in a local factory. His wife had a clerical position in the same organisation and since the job was still open for her, it had seemed appropriate,when the baby was born, for Ray to take on the childminding, housekeeping role. This had worked reasonably well although money was always tight. They had continued thus for the past 18 months during which time Jackie, Ray's wife,had been promoted. She was now earning more money. Not that Ray knew the exact details,for his wife still gave him the same amount of money to manage on as they had originally agreed. Jackie told him that she was putting the extra amount away each week as savings to secure their future.

Over the recent months, however, Jackie was often out in the evening for business meetings and she had begun to look very smart on these occasions. At weekends, when they went as a family to visit relatives, people would comment on how attractive she was, she would be lively and outgoing and Ray would feel the comparison keenly. He found he was becoming more and more introverted and even shy, with very little to talk about other than the children's progress. Things were not going very well at home either.

Just over a month before the referral, Ray had finally found proof of his suspicions that his wife was having an affair. He waited until she went to work the next day and, in a powerful rage, took a pair of scissors and cut up all the clothes in her wardrobe. The noisy scene on her return resulted in the police being called, followed by their calling the GP, a duty psychiatrist and a social worker. All of these women thought Ray's behaviour totally inexplicable and he was told he was mentally ill, given a powerful, long acting tranquilliser, taken to hospital and kept there for a week. On his return home, the community nurse referred him for social work support because she was worried about the effect of Ray's illness on the children!

This is a true story where only the gender, of course, and names of the participants have been changed. For Ray, read Jackie; for Ray's wife, read Jackie's husband. The last straw for Jackie was her husband taking his mistress on holiday back to the Caribbean island that was home for Jackie herself as well as for him, a home she had not been able to visit since she emigrated to England 12 years earlier. It was on his return from this holiday that she destroyed his clothes. She had no history of previous mental illness nor was she to display any subsequent symptoms, but notwithstanding this she was diagnosed to be suffering from schizophrenia, with her behaviour and her husband's information as the evidence cited to support this view.

Schizophrenia is a complex and controversial diagnosis. Current psychiatric diagnostic practice is based on the Present State Examination (PSE), a standardised interview, which describes a series of first rank symptoms which, when present, suggest a diagnosis of acute schizophrenia. One of these symptoms is termed 'thought insertion', the essence of which is that the person experiences thoughts 'which are not her or his own' intruding into her or his mind. We would suggest that women, who in general are socialised not to express their anger and are thus more liable than men to repress it from the conscious mind, may be at particular risk of experiencing thoughts of rage and hate as not belonging to them.

Another first rank symptom of schizophrenia is that described as 'autochthonous' delusional thought. This implies false belief or beliefs which cannot be altered by showing it/them logically to be false, which arise without prior reference and which are out of keeping with that person's culture, life experience and situation. It does not take a great stretch of the imagination here to consider that the stereotypical responses in those males involved with Jackie at the time — her husband and the white professional workers — could easily result in such a diagnosis of a woman behaving very angrily and much 'out of keeping' with her expected role.

Current thinking about the etiology of schizophrenia points towards the possibility of a genetic causative factor with social factors highly relevant in affecting its course (e.g. Gottesman and Shields, 1982, Vaughan and Leff, 1976). Psychological theories on the development of schizophrenia have emphasized the role of the family and the mother in particular, although there is little clear research evidence as yet to confirm this. A review of several studies into family interactions, identified that:

> Mothers of schizophrenics are more concerned, protective, and possibly more intrusive than control mothers both in the current situation and in their attitudes to the children before they showed signs of schizophrenia. (Hirsch and Leff, quoted in Newton, 1989: 96)

Hirsch and Leff noted that this over-protectiveness could result from having a difficult child rather than vice versa and recent analysis of a longitudinal comparison study has identified early trauma and difficult behaviour in the lives of children who later suffer what are termed schizophrenic breakdowns (Mednick, Schulsinger and Venables, 1981). It is significant, however, that the temptation to blame mother became institutionalised in the literature:

> Schizophrenogenic; Adj; applied usually to parent, typically mother whose personality and behaviour is held (by user) capable of inducing schizophrenia in her children (Rycroft, 1979).

For mental health workers looking for a more in-depth development of current thinking on the origins of schizophrenia we recommend the chapter in Jennifer Newton's book 'Preventing Mental Illness' (Newton, 1988). However, our position remains that 'labelling' people in this way can result in inappropriate interventions with serious and long lasting consequences. A too-hasty attachment of a diagnostic label can close professionals' eyes to the circumstances in women's lives which may contribute to the apparently bizarre behaviour being demonstrated. Nor in our experience are labels once made easily re-evaluated.

What is clear to us as professionals looking at responses to women in trouble is how easy it is to appreciate 'Rays' behaviour as one of appropriate anger in a situation where his feelings were not considered, where he felt undervalued and his goodwill abused. In real life, neither the male professionals involved nor perhaps Jackie herself, were in touch with her behaviour as an understandable reaction to considerable provocation, nor did they make a link back to when her problems originated in what may well have been post-puerperal depression. Instead, she was labelled psychotic and hospitalised.

The final insult to Jackie must be that her own needs did not even merit a referral for social work support aimed at preventing a further deterioration in her condition. What society was interested in was to safeguard her role as a caregiver to her children. Traditional social work responses focus primarily on the needs of the children in such cases. To this end a play group for the baby and after school activities for the older child, together with monitoring Jackie's medication, might well have been the priority of the social work intervention. However, on referral, Jackie's social worker was careful to explore the personal and social circumstances that could be contributing to her mental health problems. Together they began to understood her experience as an uncontrolled explosion of unexpressed rage and resentment which had been building up over many years.

Casework, therefore, focused on empowering Jackie to assert herself with her husband, her children, and the housing department. In consultation with the general practitioner, Jackie's medication was slowly cut down. Regular social work home visits were initiated and were followed, as her confidence grew, by supportive sessions in the social work office. These aimed at improving Jackie's self image in various ways. In subsequent joint sessions with both Jackie and her husband, the social worker encouraged Jackie to put her point of view to Ray despite his considerable hostility. The housing department were asked to repair the damp in the flat and Jackie redecorated. Through time, she sued for divorce and claimed her share of the joint savings, although sadly little remained by then to be shared. Eventually, the now single parent family moved to another flat away from the unhappy memories of the marital home and the children gradually experienced their mother in a more positive, stable and independent role.

By focusing on Jackie's needs and exploring and addressing the circumstances of her life, therefore, the worker had ultimately promoted the well-being of the children as well as producing a better role model for their own future relationships. Jackie's social worker was based in a fieldwork department of a local social services agency and whilst the origins of the department's concern, the child care, allowed for her to support Jackie and the family, Jackie's mental health could have been a low priority for another worker not so experienced or knowledgeable about mental health.

This story raises many issues, not least that of the need for mental health workers to understand some of the cultural issues impinging on this case which involved a black family being responded to by white workers. Within the National Health Service, Dr. Parimala Moodley, a black woman psychiatrist, has been instrumental in the setting up of the Maudsley Outreach Support Team, a multi-disciplinary team of doctors, community psychiatric nurses and social workers, community liaison workers, researchers and administrative staff based in Camberwell, London. A need was identified for ongoing help for people in the locality with chronic mental health problems who would normally become part of the 'revolving door' process. People are traditionally admitted in crisis, stabilised and discharged home on medication to be followed up in the outpatients department. Often they relapse as a result of the home circumstances which contributed to the stress remaining unaddressed, or as a result of insufficient follow-up support to encourage continuing medication or other forms of treatment. It was recognised that the majority of this group of people in this area were from ethnic minority backgrounds and that an off-site, intensive outreach service would be more approachable than the traditional hospital model.

The team visits discharged patients at home and asks what help the patient would like in an assessment aimed at helping to improve the quality of life. Subsequent interventions might involve help in a range of problem areas including personal counselling, family support, housing and income advice. A drop-in service is provided and the team employs a team management system so that, although each person has a key worker, she/he can usefully be seen by other members of the team in the key worker's absence. Dr. Moodley identifies the particular strength of the team as its interest in working with a generally undervalued group and its mix and balance of race and gender. Openness and sensitivity to each other in order to address the individual needs of people in a multi-cultural locality are essential and are developed through skills-sharing exercises, close supervision and a regular staff support group where issues such as stereotyping and prejudice both within the group and with patients can be explored safely.

Depression

Many young women who come into contact with the mental health system do so because they experience depression. Women describe the experience of depression in different ways:

> 'It just goes on and on. It colours everything. You feel like there is nothing you want to do, nothing seems worthwhile. In fact the whole world seems grey.'

> 'Usually if it's sunny I feel cheerful, but when I'm depressed even a beautiful sunny day feels like nothing. I just think 'so what?' I can't get excited about anything, not even a friend or a piece of cake. Nothing seems worth it. Any good feelings of pleasure of warmth seem to have gone for good. I try and imagine how I could have ever felt happy, and I can't.'

> 'It's awful but I start to hate my family. Everything they do irritates me. I just don't want anyone near me. Then I hate myself. I feel I'm no good at anything. I feel a failure. Someone can just say a little thing and it makes me cry. Anything makes me cry. When I was depressed, it was so awful, I thought I'd never get rid of it.' (Rosenthall & Greally 1988: 4)

Women may feel anxious, overly concerned about their health and have difficulty in concentrating or sleeping. They may lose their appetite, their sexual desire and become socially isolated. Negative ideas and apathy may also feature. This all contributes to an overall effect of a lowered ability or even wish to cope.

The typical response to women experiencing such distress is often to provide medication which can provide relief and relaxation in the short term, but which does not address the distress itself. This has been described as 'damping down' the distress so that it becomes more manageable both for the woman herself and for those around her (Rosenthall and Greally 1988: 13/14).

The medical diagnosis of depression is subject to almost as much controversy as that of schizophrenia. Doctors continue to debate the question of whether depression is one condition presenting in different ways or whether we should be thinking about a series of conditions. Currently doctors tend to think in terms of a continuum of depressive presentations according to the degree to which the woman's functioning is affected: from exogenous (reactive to a specific event) to endogenous (arising from within). Sometimes added to these labels are qualifying adjectives such as 'agitated' (if the woman is also displaying anxiety) or 'puerperal' (to indicate post-natal depression). 'Clinical depression' suggests a severity greater than the lay term indicating a depressed mood. 'Manic depressive psychosis' is much less common and its incidence, unlike other depressions, seems equal in both men and women. Here major swings of mood are experienced with periods of stability in between. There is evidence to suggest that genetic and biological factors contribute to the incidence of this condition as well as to severe clinical depression and this factor should not be disregarded. Most of the major research, however, has focused on psycho-social factors, some of which we discuss in our case studies. (Here also for a detailed discussion we suggest reference to Newton's book.)

Women may co-operate with the doctor's assessment that they are suffering from some sort of chemical imbalance, in other words, a physical illness. Temptingly, the medical model offers an isolated and depressed woman a sense of finally being looked after by someone who understands the problem without suggesting that some responsibility for the solution might belong with her. One in every five women take some form of tranquillisers.

Medication can have an important role to play in relieving some of the most debilitating effects of depression. But the continuing use of medication as a means of obscuring the causes of depression cannot be defended. For some women at this critical stage in their lives, objective circumstances have a large part to play. These may either be features of the experience of childbirth itself (examples can be found in Ann Oakley's book 'Women Confined'), or the circumstances women have to cope with after their child is born:

> 'My husband was around sometimes but he doesn't know much about babies and all my family are back in Africa. So I had to do everything for myself and it was hard. Before I could go out I had to get the pram and two kids down all the stairs. It was too much so I usually didn't bother. I stayed home and talked to the walls, getting more lonely and depressed.' (Quoted in Alison Corob, 1987: 60.)

But there is also a way in which our society 'disallows' certain feelings or only allows their expression in stereotypical ways which may reinforce feelings of helplessness and thus contribute to depression:

> The types of feelings we are expected to show are vulnerable ones. We often cry when we want to get angry. We express our feelings in ways which seem weak rather than strong. But whether we cry or shout, we are still liable to be labelled by men as 'hysterical' or 'over-emotional' or 'attention-seeking'. Paradoxically, to be a 'real woman' we are supposed to express feelings, but when we do so we are still likely to be put down either directly or by being ignored. (Nairne and Smith, 1984: 50.)

In a society where people tend to defend themselves from experiencing the unhappy and uncomfortable feelings that are part of the life cycle of all of us, it is easy to see why the pills that protect us from these can be so enticing. Medication may be used to obtain temporary relief, but a longer term plan should be aimed towards addressing the origins of the problems. Many women suffering from depression are able to feel sufficiently supported by counsellors or other support group members to cope with their symptoms unaided by medication. For others, particularly where the depression is too severe for them to be able to use such help, initial symptom relieving anti-depressants can work constructively with other therapeutic help aimed towards longer term readjustment. A number of studies (e.g. Holmes and Rahe, 1967, Dohrenwend 1973, Dohrenwend and Dohrenwend, 1974) have shown that events such as the death of a close family member, pregnancy, changing jobs, a child leaving home, major material loss or disappointment or even happy events, such as marriage, and family holidays, can be predictors of mental health breakdown. Brown and Harris (1978) identified a clear causal link with life events preceding the onset of depressive symptoms in the women they studied and suggested that it was the meaning of the particular losses that was important in bringing about the depression.

> 'Adaptation and accommodation to a major loss or disap-
> pointment might go on for months, if not years, perhaps
> with some element of denial and then an event, sometimes
> quite trivial, would 'break through' to underline the hope-
> lessness of the position' (Brown and Harris, ibid: 277).

This research showed women who had experienced an interruption in their care in childhood were three times as likely to be depressed as women whose parenting was 'normal'. It was the lack of care which followed the loss of a parent rather than the loss itself which was established as the important factor. Thus the possibility is that for vulnerable women the new change will echo an earlier sense of isolation and lost care. Women, stereotypically brought up to be passive, with the belief that they would never have their needs met nor, indeed, were they deserving of the love and affection they craved, might well be more vulnerable to depression for this reason. As well as the new losses involved in the changes following childbirth, the experience may also evoke the grief and distress women were not encouraged to express as infants.

Good enough mothers

The real difficulties women who are mothers face when they feel sad and angry about the care they themselves received is highlighted in Kathleen's story.

Kathleen

Kathleen was a married woman in her 20s when she was referred to the Child Guidance Service. She was the mother of three boys aged 7, 3 and 2. There had been a cot death of a girl child before the two younger boys. She had difficulty in offering consistent mothering to any of her children but her major problem was in relating to her oldest boy, David. He was not functioning well at school and, in a recent incident, Kathleen had hit him quite badly when she found him bending over the youngest boy's cot. The names of all the children were subsequently placed on the 'At Risk' register, when the two-year-old was found to have taken some of his mother's tablets.

Growing up with a father who left when she was two and a mother who beat her, Kathleen was first sent to boarding school and then ran away into care at 15. She had learnt that if you made enough fuss, you managed to get attention and this seemed to be the only way to get things done. Otherwise, speaking up normally in her family resulted in 'getting clobbered' and achieving nothing.

She carried into her contact with the professional workers her ambivalence about dependence. She wanted help from them but when she was receiving it, this would seem to reinforce a sense of her own helplessness and she would feel undermined. Thus, she would come to see her worker and overwhelm her with her volubility, one issue would merge into another and it would be difficult to contain and concentrate on anything. Then she would miss appointments or be late. Gradually, however, Kathleen began to be more focused. She allowed herself to be 'mothered' by her worker as they began to explore the important issues in a constructive way. Kathleen explored her relationship with David and worked on how she might understand his feelings when he is on the receiving end of her inconsistencies. At length, Kathleen's confidence increased to the extent that she could focus, was taking responsibility for herself and setting conditions for her husband that are acceptable to both parties. She says, 'I do now love David' and is working closely with his school where she is learning to handle him with more consistency and assertion.

Mothers are often the target of blame - by their children, by professionals, by society - for the inadequacies in their parenting. It is an impossible job to get right. Experts have been giving women different advice for years. The problem is that while they are still arguing about the best ways of child rearing, mothers only have their experiences of being mothered to draw on. The temptation in Kathleen's case was for the professionals to have gone along with Kathleen's initial wish and removed David from her care. In this instance, however, she found a worker prepared to understand her ambivalence, to reach out to the needy child inside her and, in so doing, offer Kathleen a metaphorical experience of what proper mothering could be like. Kathleen's own fears about herself as a bad mother were then explored in a way that allowed her self-confidence to grow, both for her own benefit and for her children's as well. There will still be problems for this family to surmount but her positive experience at this stage will allow Kathleen to ask for help more appropriately.

Newpin is an organisation based in London and run by mothers for mothers, which aims to intervene in the chain of isolation and destruction in families where women suffering from depression are trying to cope with young families with little support.

This project 'matches' women, putting a 'supporter' with a similar experience in touch with a new client to visit them at home and share their concerns. In this way, it is hoped the women can develop a friendship that in time will encourage the new client to use the project-based Newpin service. Here mothers with their children are offered a service that includes intensive psychotherapy, on a group and individual basis, and a crèche. They also find an opportunity to mix with other women and children and to make new friends. A member describes her initial feelings:

'I found it quite difficult because I was quite frightened
of walking through the door and seeing these people I
didn't know, so I used to beg my supporter to bring me
and to meet me, and we met on a regular basis. But after
a few months, I began to come up on my own but it was
quite frightening.'

Others who are reaching the end of a training group programme
share their feelings:

'I think once I started to use the group analysis and do
some work on myself, that was very difficult, very hard
going but I viewed myself differently afterwards. I
thought about myself much more positively and tended
not to be so negative. I think all in all at the end of that
training group the quality of my own life started to improve and subsequently, of course, Morgan's did. For the
first time in my life at the age of 26, I began to realise who
I was — "this is me, this is the person", and "this is why
I get all these bad feelings and why I don't like going in
lifts and on tubes". It's really odd; all these things that
come up for you while you're in the therapy group and
you relate them, and it just all clicks into place.'

Apart from learning about themselves, the women also discussed
their learning in other areas such as child development and asked
for more workshops on issues such as divorce and relationship
breakdowns and how these affect children.

A research project studying some of the women from the over
500 families who had used the Newpin project, found that nearly
half came from broken homes, 40% had at least one change of main
person looking after them in their childhood, 28% had been
physically injured by their main carer, 13% had been physically
abused and a third had been in care. 65% had treatment of some
kind for mental 'ill health' and 53% had mental health problems
lasting for at least two years (Pound *et al* 1985).

A similar organisation offering a voluntary befriending scheme
and intensive, well-structured health visiting for mothers of young

children in disadvantaged families is Homestart, a community based organisation funded by the Department of Health and local charities in Leicester. Here volunteers on a 'mum to mum' basis aim to build up the mother's self-confidence, help her find stimulating things to do with her children and generally gain a sense of pleasure and fulfilment from her role. Both of these organisations are considerably less expensive than the cost of traditional social services involvement as well as providing a self-help model which directly challenges the sense of helplessness which is so contributory to depression (Seligman, 1975).

Newpin and Homestart have organisational structures specifically aimed to encourage and empower both their users and their staff. Mental health workers in more hierarchical settings might look to specific interventions they themselves can use in their client's best interests.

Carol

Carol had a history of depression that went back to a time of many changes. She was married at 19, lived at home with her parents and during a two-year period had a child, lost her mother, was kicked out of the family home subsequent to a row with her father, lived in temporary accommodation, was rehoused and had a second child. Her mother had died rather suddenly of cancer and it was not until eight months later that Carol shed her first tears. She was on various anti-depressants for a large part of the following nine years, had some periods of in-patient treatment and offers of counselling at the hospital as well as field social work support which she felt she had not been able to use. At that time, she said, she felt unable to say very much.

Her background was a childhood marred by continuous marital disharmony. Her father was a compulsive gambler and mother took control of the finances. The father often attempted to cheat mother about money and in their negotiations and arguments he would resort to violence. Carol remembered a little figurine of two lovers on the television set that she would turn to face the wall when these arguments were in process. Her mother had 'bad nerves' all her life and Carol blamed father for hastening her death by his violence.

Two years before she asked for help to deal with her underlying problems, Carol had begun to drink. She would do this on her way home from work and doing so enabled her to get in touch with the feelings she could not otherwise express. They were mostly feelings of anger towards her husband and at times were very violent. She used to kick the walls and hurt her hands but never actually hurt anyone else. Her husband seemed to understand some of the things she tried to tell him but they had managed to resolve the problem by seeing very little of each other. He was now on night work and she concentrated on her mothering role when at home and now, as her daughters were growing towards independence, Carol herself was feeling she had never really had a life. She described herself as always anxiously trying to adapt herself to what other people seemed to want and having no sense of her own needs or rights.

The hospital social worker at this stage offered Carol a programme of short-term therapy to address her problems . This model of therapy involves the client in conjunction with the worker in an essentially problem-solving model of work, although the method of work also uses many psychoanalytic concepts. Together the two women worked out a focus for their work that described Carol's central dilemma as follows:

'I live my life as if, in relationships, I must be either passively giving in to others, or overwhemlingly destructive.'

They agreed to challenge Carol's view of her options, and in the therapy, Carol had the opportunity to test out whether her view of the world until now, that relationships with people were so two-dimensional, was correct. To do so she learned to allow the therapist to care for her in a way she had never thought her mother was strong enough to do. Early on in their time together she began to complete the mourning for her mother, explored her anger with her and then acted out her rage at what she saw as the social worker's inflexibility and lack of understanding of her needs. This, interestingly, took the form of being too 'ill' to attend the session and when she came to the next one she spoke movingly of the loneliness that 'changing' seemed to be bring with it. She sensed her children and husband combining to keep her as she had always been and how threatened they seemed to be when she was more assertive with them. Carol persevered with her new behaviour as her understanding of the self-perpetuating patterns of her life so far grew.

As the therapy ended, Carol told the worker of her determination to see things through. Now that she had started, she saw no way of going back. She was not prepared to be a mother to her husband as well as the children but wanted him to begin to take greater responsibility in the family. She was more assertive with her children and began to allow them the independence they were seeking.

She had valued the therapy and admitted to disappointment that things still remained to be tackled as well as a sense of real loss of her relationship with a 'good enough' carer. In the last session, she openly mourned both her mother and her valued social worker.

Carol's social worker offered Carol therapy as part of a research project based at a London teaching hospital where a time-limited, integrated method of cognitive analytic therapy was being offered as part of the National Health Service provision in the hospital's catchment area. The strengths of this intervention are obvious in terms of empowerment. Carol had made sense of her life and future in the light of early experiences that seemed to offer very limited options for her as a woman, as a wife and mother. In her childhood, her father was the abusive and her mother abused and unassertive. Carol's very appropriate anger seemed dangerous to her and she feared that expressing it would make her like her father. She distanced herself from these feelings both unconsciously and consciously in collusion with the doctors who continued to prescribe anti-depressant medication for nine years.

When her own daughters began to remind her of herself and her sister in the years when they witnessed the marital fighting, Carol's control broke down. She was fortunate to have access to a service that allowed her to explore her feelings appropriately and to make sense of much that had happened to her. Her changing outlook upset the equilibrium, unsatisfactory though it was, with her husband and children and the marriage was unlikely to survive. A considerable change for the better, however, was that, at follow up, she was much more confident, had a better job and was herself a more positive role model for her children. The hope is also that the old abusing/abused pattern may not necessarily be the model for the children's future relationships.

This model of short-term therapy, provided by a social worker in this instance, is intensive and thus provides early pain relief, can be used in individual therapy as in this case or in groups, and has been shown to be successful both in the short and long term in many settings, both statutory and voluntary, medical and non-medical (Ryle, 1990). It can enable the woman herself to take more control of her own life and can help to prevent a repetition of dysfunctional behaviour in her children. Cognitive analytic therapy does require a form of specialist training, albeit shorter than a traditional psychotherapy training, for the basically qualified mental health worker to be able to work in this way. As described in the section on groupwork with sexually abused children, however, we see such an input as highly preventive, more empowering and less oppressive than some other psychotherapy models and, in this instance, equally resource efficient thus meeting organisational needs in settings such as the National Health Service and social services.

Again, as with Jackie and Kathleen, the social worker focused her work on Carol's needs rather than monitoring child care as a priority and this raises the question of accountability. In the event that the children had been hurt in any way, questions might well have been asked about the responsibility of the social worker. Social workers are constantly placed in the invidious position of attempting to meet all needs as well as satisfy the public wish to pretend that all is well in our stereotypical family. By going along with this, they leave themselves at risk of being blamed when the evidence that this is not the case asserts itself. Social workers and the caring professions generally need to avoid colluding with the belief that they can be all things to all people. Perhaps it will then be more possible to empower the women they work with to assert themselves more appropriately.

In the final chapter of this book we suggest how some of the organisational changes currently taking place within social care agencies in the United Kingdom may serve to bring about a separation between child care and adult responsibilities. This may provide a structure in which focusing on adult mental health needs separately from children's needs can be legitimated.

Summary

Women's experiences of the world differ radically from men's yet this difference has not been sufficiently acknowledged by families and professionals alike. The reality of the experience of motherhood and childbirth can be very different from the images of happy families with which young women are still presented. Combining work with family responsibilities can create additional stresses if responsibilities within the family group do not change. Professional responses often imply that it is perfectly appropriate for adult women to be passive, dependent and unable to cope yet at the same time the myth of the all-providing wife and mother who should be able to meet all the family's needs in a self-sacrificing way remains. The case studies quoted here have shown women's frustration as well as their temptation to co-operate with services that reinforce their helplessness. Initiatives that have questioned women's passivity are shown to have much to offer to promote change. Counselling and psychotherapy, women supporting each other be it individually or in groups, are all areas where women are now finding support which can lead to positive changes in their lives. Those working with women experiencing mental distress may have to help them identify how they may be trying to live their lives in response to stereotypes which prevent them from understanding their own needs or which cause self-blame because the reality does not live up to expectations. Women becoming mothers have to deal with both the very personal changes motherhood brings as well as the awesome images of Good Mother and Bad Mother which have such powerful connotations in our society.

4. MID-LIFE AND EARLY OLD AGE:
'Invisibility'

'.... the different life experiences of men and women do
not magically disappear with age ....' (Sheila Peace)

'A man is as old as he's feeling, a woman as old as she
looks' (Oxford Dictionary of Quotations)

Our discussions in the previous two chapters have started to
demonstrate the connectedness between experiences taking place at
one time and emotional and behavioural responses which may result
later. Women growing older may bring with them emotional distress
experienced when they were younger and which still has not been
resolved. For others, mid-life and early old age may bring the need
for new adjustments which previous experiences have left them
ill-equipped to handle.

Mid-life can be a time of the greatest creativity when
professional ambitions have been achieved and children are
becoming more independent, leaving space for their parents' own
needs to be pursued and for marriages to be reassessed. But it is
also a time when other options are narrowing. The psychoanalyst
Erikson (1963) challenged the narrow focus of intrapsychic theories
of development by stressing the interplay between life stages and
the shaping processes of social settings. Whilst he also lacked a
gender perspective, we believe his description of the conflict of
middle age as that of generativity versus stagnation is helpful and
very relevant to women.

Mid-life may be a time when increasing physical limitations start
to become evident. In official statistics a woman of 60 is elderly
because that is the official retirement age (although this is now
being challenged). A man is not similarly 'old' until he reaches 65.
But chronological age has very little to do with personal experiences
of feeling old or being defined by others as elderly. Some studies of
old people in black communities have taken 55 as the starting point
of old age because the harsh life experiences of many black people
mean that ageing takes place earlier.

For women who are mothers mid-life is a time when they may start to be aware that their children are leading more interesting lives than themselves. No longer are their children dependent, not even for lifts to meet friends or go to a rock concert. They are starting to go to college, get jobs, move in with friends, get married and separate their lives from those of their parents. Mid-life for such women can offer a longed-for freedom from sexual and domestic responsibilities, a new adolescence even. The other side of the coin for many women, however, is the loss of a role for which they can see no easily found replacement.

For women who are wives, relationships with their husbands may have to adjust as they become a couple again rather than parents in a family household. And every woman faces an essentially personal transition, the menopause — 'the change' as it is sometimes known. No longer is the ability to bear children a part of her identity. If she has children this may represent a loss of something which has been a fundamental part of her life; for women who have not borne children, whether by choice or not, the menopause represents the door finally closing on the possibility of being mothers themselves. However comfortable women may have been with their decisions in this area, it is likely that feelings of loss, whether it be of career or motherhood, will be revived at this time.

Women who are daughters may find this a time when they have to decide whether they should give up work to care for an ageing parent. Clare Ungerson (Ungerson, 1987) in her study of informal carers explores how women are 'available' for caring at different stages in their life cycle than are men. Whilst

'Full time paid work almost always acts as a buffer between the social and family circumstances of a man and his availability for caring,' (p.65)

for women, child care responsibilities and responsibilities for caring for elderly relatives are likely to merge:

'Thus, just as they were reaching the point in the life cycle where most women would expect to be able to make somewhat self-indulgent plans for their own future, these women were facing an indefinite period of caring.' (p.66)

At a time when men are likely to be at the peak of their careers, a working woman may feel both internal and external pressures to forsake her career in order to become a full-time carer.

Fransella and Frost (1977) consider the limited research which focuses on how women see themselves as they grow older. The fact that most research concentrates on women as childbearers and young mothers demonstrates what it is about women that is seen to be of interest or importance. The contemporary focus on women as informal carers makes a similar point. Women's needs and concerns become visible when they relate to their roles as caregivers and thus become significant from the perspective of social policy and social welfare. As mothers, they may be subject to scrutiny to ensure that their mothering is acceptable, as carers of elderly or disabled relatives their needs may be acknowledged to ensure that they can continue in that role. Stresses associated with caring are increasingly being recognised and some help is being offered to women whose emotional distress derives from that. We would not in any way want to detract from this, but we also think it is important to acknowledge that the women concerned receive help because they are carers. Women who are not caregivers, or who are no longer in that position, may find it rather harder to be offered help in their own right.

The 'invisibility' of women in mid-life is summed up in a quote which Fransella and Frost found in an unpublished manuscript. It comes from an interview with a sculptor who was asked whether he ever made busts of middle-aged women:

> 'I've tried, but it is very difficult. Middle-aged women seem to have no image. They hide behind make-up and sweet and youthful manners. They bind up their breasts, and try to hide it if the hips are too wide. Sometimes, when they get lost in thought, one notices that they really are grandmothers. The old woman is much more interesting. An old wrinkled face may be very beautiful. And the old woman possesses an image: the greatest artists have painted her. Looking at her, one is reminded of The Grandmother, taking care of all the children that surround her. Middle-aged woman is difficult, with lines in her face which she tries to hide. But most important: she has no

image.' (Sandsberg, 1976, quoted in Fransella and Frost 1977,: 113–114.)

She has no image because there is no role which provides a positive statement of what a woman in mid-life has to offer. Stereotypical images are almost entirely negative: the middle-aged frump discarded by her husband for an attractive younger woman, the menopausal woman with her hot flushes, the ageing spinster who was never able to get her man. It is perhaps not surprising that depression is a common experience for women as they grow older.

The prescription of tranquillisers to women increases as they get older. In part this is because they may be prescribed as sleeping pills. What starts as an aid to sleeping at a time of severe distress or depression, following bereavement for example, may continue into long term prescribing. Such a response can numb reactions, but act to avoid the need to understand the response to loss. A woman during mid-life may experience multiple losses, sometimes at the same time:

> 'In common with many women, my menopause coincided with the death of my mother and the emergent adolescence/adulthood of the children I have parented. Both partings were painful and the loss of my mother a particularly protracted agony. The emotional and mental confusion at these events was hard to disentangle from the effects of my body's journey from pre- to post-menopause.' (Robertson, 1983).

Not all women bringing up children are heterosexual and it would be wrong to assume that a lessening of childcare responsibilities has no significance for some lesbian women. For all women, mid-life may be a time to take action at last or not at all, to fulfil themselves in ways that seemed impossible before, perhaps in terms of pursuing relationships hitherto felt as unacceptable both to themselves and those around them. But lesbian women may be at a particular disadvantage in situations where a marital relationship would seem to provide rights. For example, rights relating to hospital care of the loved partner or provision for the distribution of a deceased partner's property or, indeed, even being seen as bereaved at all.

There are few comfortably attainable successful role models for women at this stage of their lives. The role model of the powerful woman provided by former Prime Minister Margaret Thatcher served both to stereotype as 'wet' any concern with caring, and to assert with great force the moral superiority of the independent (preferably wealthy) individual over interdependent, supporting relationships. That provided by women such as Joan Collins and Jane Fonda seems both practically impossible to achieve for the majority of women, and to emphasise a denial of the ageing process.

If the role of caregiver is not required, then women have to seek some form of occupation to fill their time, in some cases for the first time, in others by attempting to return to an occupation which was left many years ago. Whether it be voluntary or paid employment, women starting jobs at this stage in their lives are unlikely to have the status of men whose career has progressed unbroken. Employment may well involve again a supportive role, caring for others but now in the workplace as a secretary or a social work assistant. Rarely are the talents of women who have spent many years managing and organising families recognised for the valuable management skills they actually are, a fact which must be a considerable lost resource to a country suffering from a lack of skilled managers.

Even feminism has tended to neglect older women's issues and we believe this is in part a result of ambivalent feelings which many women have about their own mothers. Women who regard themselves as feminists may have a tendency to blame their mothers for what they see as collusion with male values or as simply failing to provide them with a positive and strong role model. Shere Hite's study of daughters' views of their mothers provides evidence of this:

> 'The majority of women have distressed and confused feelings about their mothers; 73% feel a very deep love and ties, but also a great disappointment or anger about their mothers' subservience, 'passivity' — or even 'cowardice' — in the face of their husbands' authority.'(Hite, 1990: 15.)

One woman's view quoted by Hite describes graphically the ambivalence in her attitude to her mother and the fear and resentment felt when recognising her mother's qualities in herself:

> 'My mother is the world's greatest victim. She never took control of her life . . . . Am I like my mother, I never wanted to be like her, hate it when I am . . . .when I can be the 'victim' of life, when I get to needy, when I have high approval needs. I resent her passing those things on to me.' (Hite, 1990: 15.)

Women as Carers

We have noted that mid-life may be a time when women take on new caring roles. The decision to take on the role of carer for an elderly or disabled relative may not always be a conscious one. Women may feel it is their duty, or others may assume that it is and behave in such a way as to leave her with little real choice. Caring for an elderly or disabled relative can be a source of both physical and mental stress. A survey of sole carers carried out by the 'Crossroads' Care Attendant organisation provides typical findings: 81% of those responding to a question about ill health caused by caring said that it had had an adverse affect on their health. Illnesses reported varied from stress-related asthma to ulcers, heart conditions, mental health problems, and muscle, shoulder and back problems, 57% gave a positive response to the statement 'I feel like crying,' 49% said 'yes' to the statement: 'I am often at breaking point' and 35% agreed that 'I feel totally isolated' (Crossroads, 1990).

The need for emotional support, respite and practical help for carers is increasingly being recognised by both statutory and voluntary agencies (see for example Twigg, Atkin and Perring, 1990). Such services both directly and indirectly assist the mental health of those taking on this role. But what happens when the caring stops?

Marjorie

Marjorie had been a carer for much of her life, both at home for her parents where, as they grew old, she had taken on a full time caring role unsupported by her two brothers, and at work where she had been a highly valued 'Girl Friday'.

Loss may be accompanied by feelings of guilt. Marjorie, now 55 years old, described to us her reaction when her mother died:

> 'I felt a bit lost, guilt, if only . . . . these sorts of things. I should have given up work a long time before I did . . . .'

But alongside the loss of a loved mother and the feelings of guilt were other feelings of loss. We asked Marjorie what was the worst thing she felt after her mother died:

> 'The actual loss of her physically because I'd done so much for her and had so much contact with her physically - made her look nice and bought her clothes and dressed her. And then there was nothing. I remember standing in the front room, not long afterwards, after the funeral and it seemed as though it was the whole world and there was nothing there, just isolation and I did pray to die because she was not there and I wanted to be with her. And the whole routine had collapsed. There was nothing to get up for in the morning, she wasn't there to be seen to. I did enjoy doing it once I'd accepted and made the decision for myself to do it — I felt it was like another career.'

Women 'freed' from the role of carer thus do not always experience this as a liberation. Losing the caring role may leave nothing; for the mother because that is all her adult life has contained, for the daughter because other roles have been given up in order to take on responsibility for caring for parents. Marjorie at 55 is bravely planning to start a college course to update her office skills which had become outdated in the time she had been caring for her mother and father who had also recently died. But her confidence was extremely low, she rarely went out and had little contact with other people. It is not certain that she would be able to complete that course without support. She had rejected the offer of tranquillisers after her mother had died. She had benefited from going to a carers group both whilst she was caring for her mother and for some time after she had died, but when that group stopped,

'because there just wasn't a call for it',

she was left alone at considerable risk of isolation and depression. She would not be a priority for social care for any statutory agency, but her profound unhappiness and suppressed anger at her experience of life suggest a level of need for help that it would be hard to measure against the needs of more obviously 'mentally ill' women.

A few women are fortunate to find their way to a service which attempts to meet their needs effectively. Josie's route was through a physical illness.

Josie

Josie, 48 years old, became severely depressed following a mastectomy. Traditionally a 'carer', Josie, the middle of three daughters in her family of origin, had a history of looking after a mentally disordered father, a disabled sister and more recently a somewhat fragile husband and three children of their own. In conjunction with the social worker who offered her cognitive analytic therapy (as described in Chapter Three), Josie identified the ways she had learned best to manage in her life. Relationships for her, as for many women, seemed to pose the dilemma:

'Either cared for like a regressed baby or crossly caring
for others showing what good care should be'.

In other words, Josie had no model of asking for help or receiving it in a way that did not involve her or others in feeling dependent and helpless. Thus her mode of coping was (like her mother) as 'superwoman', managing everything and everyone at considerable cost to her own needs. She finally got the rest and attention she never otherwise received only when she was seriously ill and manifestly incapable of looking after others.

With her social worker, in therapy, Josie is now learning to claim her share of care from others and gaining self-respect in ways less punishing and detrimental to both her physical and mental health. Both Josie and Marjorie point to the need for mental health workers to help women in mid-life to assert their own needs. For Josie this was primarily in the form of learning how to receive care for herself, whilst for Marjorie the need is for someone to provide her with companionship and support as she makes her way into the outside world again.

The outcomes of loss

Loss and change in later life can re-evoke the feelings attached to our earliest experiences of loss and separation from the important caring figures on which our survival seemed to depend. Bowlby suggested that grief often surfaces as the underlying cause of mental disorder:

> 'Clinical experience and a reading of the evidence leave little doubt of the truth of the main proposition — that much psychiatric illness is an expression of pathological mourning — or that such illness includes many cases of anxiety state, depressive illness, and hysteria and also more than one kind of character disorder' (Bowlby, 1980: 23).

Hysteria was perhaps the original archetypal 'female malady'. Ehrenreich and English (1979) describe it as having 'put the doctors on the spot' (p.137) because having claimed it as a disease, their professional self-esteem demanded that they find an organic cause for it. Elaine Showalter describes it as the disorder 'most strongly identified with the feminist movement' because:

81

'Doctors had noticed that hysteria was apt to appear in young women who were especially rebellious. F.C. Skey, for example, had observed that his hysterical patients were likely to be more independent and assertive than normal women, exhibiting more than usual force and decision of character, of strong resolution, fearless of danger. Donkin too had seen among his patients a high percentage of unconventional women — artists and writer.' (Showalter, 1987: 145.)

It remains a controversial diagnostic term. Rycroft (1979) has identified its use to describe: (a) conditions characterised by the presence of physical symptoms, (b) the absence of physical signs or any evidence of physical pathology and (c) behaviour suggesting the symptoms fulfil some psychological function. The main qualities apparent in the person's behaviour are described as dependency, self-interest and emotionality. Feminist therapists in the main reject the idea of an hysterical personality type as this has been used largely in a fashion that has been denigrating to women. Certainly Greenspan, describing what she calls the 'Diagnostic Detective Game' she learned during her medical training, makes some telling observations:

'Educated, middle-class male patients were invariably diagnosed as obsessive-compulsive personalities. Women were most often hysterics (though more highly educated or male-identified women tended also to be diagnosed as obsessives). And working class people, male or female, black or white, were almost always borderline personalities.' (Greenspan, 1983: 53.)

The notion of hysteria derived from the ancient Greeks who applied the term solely to diseases of women and Plato's definition of an hysteric was of a woman possessed with a disturbed uterus which was wandering around loose and presumably causing untold chaos! As described earlier, the numbers of men presenting with 'hysterical' symptoms after battle experiences caused some psychiatric rethinking but it is not until relatively recently that the psychoanalytic textbooks have contained a rather different explanation:

> 'Women suffer these afflictions or behave in this fashion not because of anything inherent in their nature. Rather they are prone to hysteria because of cultural and environmental forces [that] men have produced, or rather have invented, the myth of a unique femininity'. (Chodoff, (1982: 564.)

Chambless and Goldstein (1980) support this view by identifying the fact that women defined as hysterics rely on the repression and denial of a range of feelings. They suggest that such a style may be learned when a child is regularly punished for the expression of strong feelings. This would tend to coincide with the stereotypical female upbringing already identified. Women who have not been encouraged to be competent, assertive, self-reliant individuals are likely to feel helpless in the face of stressful situations. Similarly, if they have been taught not to face and deal with fearful experiences but to depend on others to address them, the development of inappropriate anxiety is understandable. Is it purely coincidence that, alongside the waning of hysteria as a diagnosis for women as feminist pressure against it grows, the diagnosis of borderline personality increases in frequency?

In ancient times, hysteria was treated by fumigating the vulva of the victim with pleasant fragrances while applying noxious odours to the nose. This procedure was designed to drive the roaming uterus away from its resting place and to entice it back to its proper site! (Veith, 1965.) In studies in more recent times, women patients diagnosed as suffering from hysteria were found to have had a high frequency of gynaecological surgery (Lazare & Klerman, 1968; Winokur & Leonard 1963). which leaves us wondering if modern practices have indeed changed that much in terms of understanding and efficacy!

Lily's problems described below might in another setting have been medically diagnosed as agoraphobia. This condition, which can leave the sufferer fearful not only of 'open spaces' as the definition implies but also of trains, buses, supermarkets, crowds, and public places, is accompanied by considerable anxiety and often attacks. These attacks seem to come out of the blue and can involve difficulty in breathing, racing heart beat, faintness, and a desire to scream, run or urinate. Women form a large percentage of agoraphobia sufferers and their lives can be drastically restricted by the experience, the common theme of which seems to be a fear of any situation where escape to safe surroundings or to the support of a known and trusted other person could be hindered.

Lily

Lily, now in her mid-50s, started being 'ill' after the death of the man she worked with when she was in her mid-30s. At first she thought it was nerves. People kept saying, 'Lily is frightened to go out, she's got nerves'. Nobody asked what was wrong with her, why she was feeling like that, not even the General Practitioner who gave her tranquillisers. There was a suggestion though that it might be her age, the start of the menopause. Her 'nerves' got worse so Lily took more and more tranquillisers which were at least calming her down. But 'also it confused your mind'. Repeat prescriptions were given for Lily to pick up at the surgery without her needing to see the doctor. Lily says, 'I do keep things in. If people don't ask me, I don't tell. You feel you're causing trouble' but in reality Lily was frightened to go outside her front door, in case she wouldn't come home again, like the man who died. Later, as the full-time carer, first for her disabled mother then for her father, Lily became increasingly house-bound, suffered panic attacks when stressed and, despite various in-patient spells, is only recently at age 55 beginning to live a qualitatively improved life. This improvement she relates to a more interested woman General Practitioner and the support of the woman counsellor in the local drop-in centre.

Here Lily's needs for a 'secure base' and an opportunity to look at her relationships with the significant figures in her early life have allowed her to gain sufficient confidence to contemplate offering support to others as a volunteer worker at the centre.

Chambless and Goldstein emphasise the quality of 'anxious attachment' many phobia sufferers carry and suggest that onset of much phobic behaviour, anxiety or hysteria can emerge at times when separation or the threat of change and loss occurs and the mourning process is not properly recognised or worked through.

We believe such conditions are much more likely to exist for a woman in a society which values women first and foremost for their caring abilities, and which sees women's needs as essentially undifferentiated from those of men and children. Winnicott described the initial merging of the boundaries between mother and child which allows the mother to understand and address her new baby's needs and then gradually to let go in order in order that the child might develop her/his own identity. If mothers are blamed either for being 'over-possessive' or for being insufficiently controlling of their children, the development of extreme anxiety is an unsurprising outcome.

It has taken a feminist perspective to draw the parallels between the development of women's political consciousness and psychoanalytic accounts of the separation/individuation process, Ernst (Ernst, 1987,) confirms the need for 'constant awareness of the way in which the external world may reinforce the woman's own fears of change'. Whilst boys have a separated father to identify with and can also hope to grow up and have another woman to nurture them, for girls 'adaptation to a heterosexual society appears to mean a choice between replacing being nurtured by becoming a nurturer'. (p.98)

Services aimed specifically at women in mid-life are few and far between. Without a specific role to perform for society, women become invisible and a low priority for service intervention. One of the few organisations that does the majority of its work with women in mid - and later life is Cruse, the national organisation for people who have been bereaved. Their statistics remind us that there are currently more than 3 million widows in Britain, compared with 750,000 widowers, 1 woman in 7 is a widow and that every day 500 wives become widows.

Cruse offers help to bereaved people to work through the grieving process supported by trained volunteers. This organisation, now thirty years old, was established at a time when little attention was paid to the needs of bereaved people to work through to a healthy completion the necessary tasks of grieving for their loved ones and then moving on. Our sense is that the work of this organisation, amongst others, has led to the acceptance of part extent that in the aftermath of recent major tragedies such as the Zeebrugge ferry disaster, the King's Cross fire and the Lockerbie air crash, public and governmental support has been available to assist in the provision of bereavement counselling to grieving families but we believe there is a long way to go before service provision to the bereaved is provided in a way that enables this stage to be healthily left behind in due course.

The mourning process has four stages:
— Acceptance of loss
— Experiencing the pain associated with the loss
— Adjustment to an environment in which the deceased is absent
— Reinvesting emotional energy into new relationships, and grief counselling aims at facilitating this process. As with other states, in grief there is what could be described as a continuum of reactions, from normal to abnormal, and our concern would be aroused by the intensity or the duration of a reaction rather than to the presence or absence of any one symptom.

An abnormal grief reaction which might well contribute to future mental health problems would be one which was not satisfactorily resolved and continued for many years. Similarly, a delayed, inhibited grief reaction, or one that is masked in a physical symptom, can result in conditions that can be diagnosed as mental disorder. Lily's story above might well have been identified as an exaggerated reaction to the death of a work colleague and therapy at that stage, aimed at identifying feelings related to this and other earlier separations might have enabled her to gain more control of her life much earlier.

Mental health workers involved with women at this stage of their lives would do well to ensure that counselling and therapy focus on issues of separation and loss deriving from early experiences of relationships as well as contemporary experiences. This should include the loss of the counselling relationship. Many workers, otherwise, find themselves constantly needing to deal with recurring problems presented by women with whom they have unsuccessfully tried to complete programmes of counselling. The time-limited, cognitive analytic model, described previously, deals with loss throughout the process of the involvement, in that the date for the last meeting is known from the very beginning. This allows both client and therapist to explore issues of anger, sadness (for both of them), of 'wanting more than is available', during the course of their involvement, rather than leaving it to be acted out afterwards. A feminist mental health practice needs to go beyond helping women to adjust to loss. It also needs to be capable of empowering women to develop newly independent lives based on an awareness of their individual needs which may have been repressed during years of caring for and supporting others. Survivors groups may be important as a source of support and a safe environment within which to test out new assertiveness before moving out into more heterogeneous settings.

Long-term or severe mental health problems

After the age of 35 the proportion of female to male admissions to psychiatric hospitals starts to change and the proportion of formal admissions of women increases with each age band – in 1986 65% of formal admissions between 55 and 64 were women. It is probably safe to assume, therefore, that many women experience some form of mental distress for the first time at this stage in their lives. Alongside our concern with women like Marjorie and Lily, for whom changes during this phase of life cause emotional distress, is that we are also concerned with women who are growing older and who are already experiencing some form of mental disorder.

The disorder most commonly associated with women during their mid-life is depression: 29% of all women aged 45–54 first admitted to psychiatric hospital in 1986 had a diagnosis of depressive disorder and 31% of those aged 55–64 had a similar diagnosis. In both instances this was the single biggest diagnostic category. However, in the study of referrals to social workers under the Mental Health Act the diagnosis applied to the biggest single number of women in the 55–64 age group was schizophrenia (Barnes, Bowl and Fisher, 1990); 33.5% of women had a diagnosis of schizophrenia compared with 28% of depression. In addition 25%

of the women had a diagnosis of affective or some other form of psychosis.

As we have already said, we do not believe that diagnoses are in themselves the most helpful way of thinking about these women's needs for help. However, the women who have been diagnosed in this way are likely to have been experiencing fairly severe forms of mental distress which, in this instance, had caused someone to consider that they should be compulsorily detained in hospital. Some of these women will have had many experiences of entering psychiatric hospitals either voluntarily or under compulsion. Their 'illness' may have become a part of their identity and have had a considerable impact on the way in which they have been able to live their lives:

Janet

Janet, now in her early 50s, has been a patient in a large psychiatric hospital on the south coast for the last 25 years. Currently, as part of the effort to close down these large institutions, Janet is living in a bungalow within the hospital grounds which is identified as being for those patients who 'can't be let out'. The medical staff speak of Janet as a 'burnt out schizophrenic' and her behaviour as having much in common with the other patients in this unit. She seems to have little personal regard for herself or others. She often appears dirty or unkempt. Seemingly not knowing how to communicate with others effectively, Janet will come too close or stand too far away. Other times she can be unapproachable or sometimes she will just yell. In general, she doesn't seem to value any of the social norms adhered to in the wider society. She will urinate or defecate in unconventional areas and although there is no evidence that she has ever committed any criminal offence, it seems from the way she, and her fellow patients, are regarded and treated that society seems very fearful indeed of what, given the freedom, she just might do.

Her story gives us another insight into society's inability to tolerate women whose behaviour challenges our expectations of them. Her first admission took place following a marital row. She had left home, leaving her husband looking after their three small children. Seemingly unable to cope, he committed suicide, having first killed the children. Within a few weeks of this tragedy, Janet's GP diagnosed depression and within months she was admitted to hospital with a diagnosis of schizophrenia, the case notes stating she was 'still going on about the children!' Currently, the hospital doctors and nursing staff monitor her eating, her sleeping, her behaviour and her medication. The tragedy seems forgotten. From the immediacy of the diagnoses of mental disorder and the seeming irritation in the notes, we can but conclude that sympathetic, therapeutic attempts to help her deal with the trauma she suffered remain still outstanding.

Betty also appears to defy the social convention of womanhood:

Betty

Betty is now 48. In her life she has been a mother, a wife and has worked as a hotel receptionist. She has also been a hospital in-patient for the last 20 years including one spell in a secure hospital. Her diagnosis is 'manic-depressive', she dresses in black, spits and swears and is very offensive to male staff members. She refuses medication, is considered 'promiscuous', and 'a difficult patient whose only interest is in smoking, sex and cups of tea'.

According to her sister, Betty was an open, friendly little girl, apparently normal in every way, despite the fact that her mother had a history of identified mental disorder. She was first admitted to hospital in her 20s when she appears to have been suffering from post-natal depression after the birth of her second child. She complained at the time that her husband was unpleasant to her, keeping her short of money and going out every evening. He certainly refused to visit her in hospital or to bring the children to see her and indeed he quickly developed another liaison shortly after her admission. He was known sometimes to leave the children alone in the house when he was out in the evenings visiting his new woman friend.

As time went on, Betty seemed to get no better. She was constantly asking after the children and was angry that nothing seemed to be done to respond to her wish to see them. She became gradually more estranged from her family. One day, she absconded, took the keys to an empty house from an estate agent and moved herself and her children into it. Her behaviour was described as dangerous, bizarre, self-seeking, violent. Eventually, her behaviour becoming so difficult for the staff to tolerate, she was sent to a secure unit where not surprisingly she started 'behaving well' but quickly reverted to her angry, rejecting behaviour on her return.

Betty remains in a long-stay unit in the north of England, for people not well enough to be considered for care in the community. Yet the consultant is 'not convinced she is psychotic, more that she is simply immoral and a bad influence'. She has not yet been given that other classically stereotypical gender biased diagnosis — nymphomania!

Women in mid-life whose mental disorder is deeply rooted may have little control over their own lives:

Nancy

Nancy is 53, with a diagnosis of manic depression going back 20 years. She has been a patient continually since 1984 and is detained under Section 3 of the Mental Health Act 1983. Because of this when she goes home she is not discharged but is considered to be on extended leave. The reason for this seems to be that when she 'relapses' or her husband reaches a point where he can no longer cope with her, she can be readmitted to hospital without a reassessment.

There are clearly severe marital problems. Nancy's husband is described by the staff nurse as a man used to having his own way and difficult to deal with. Once Nancy was out shopping with a friend and, on returning later than expected, she found her husband had called the police to find her and ask for her to be readmitted!

Nancy says no one talks to her about the type of support she needs when she leaves hospital. She once went for two years without tablets because she so badly wanted to help herself. Nancy recognises that when she is in a manic phase, she is over-active and needs to learn how to control that. She has tried to find constructive ways of managing this herself but is not given any professional assistance. What is offered is a monthly visit from a community psychiatric nurse who gives her an injection and 'has a cup of coffee'. A social worker used to visit but he talked to her husband, rather than Nancy, so she asked him not to call any more. She has a day centre place once a week but 'all they do is sit and knit'.

Clearly, Nancy is receiving a professional response aimed at managing her difficulties rather than intervention. Her liberty is now very much in her husband's hands, a fact which can but adversely affect both Nancy's self-confidence and any hope of a marital relationship based on mutual respect. Nancy has been identified as 'the delinquent' with no attempt being made to address the joint contribution to stress in the relationship which must affect her progress. Nobody is listening to her!

Both Betty and Janet are also in situations where their mental disorder is being 'managed', not always very successfully. The pain and loss which each has experienced have become hidden and their identities are now defined by the behaviour which overlays their distress.

We can only suggest that the staff who provided the initial diagnoses were either insensitive to that pain, insufficiently supported to deal with the enormity of it, or could see only the aggression of the defensive behaviour of these women. Whilst we would not presume to suggest that all these women needed was grief counselling, an early therapeutic response based on an exploration of the way in which they made attachments to other people in their lives could have helped them understand something about their experience. This might have contributed towards a better understanding of their behaviour both by the women concerned and those attempting to help them as well as assisted them to avoid the tendency to make inappropriate attachments in the future.

Joy Dalton, Consultant Psychiatrist at the Whittington and Friern Barnet Hospitals in north London, emphasises the importance of teaching mental health professionals to consider issues of women's experience within society at all stages of their work. Assumptions about how emotional problems arise inevitably colour the way in which questions are asked during initial history taking, as well as at later stages in a woman's psychiatric career. Dalton teaches the need to ask questions about possible sexual and physical violence, and of trying to understand what might have affected a woman who perceives and experiences herself in a negative way.

Her model of a gender sensitive assessment and treatment plan would include the following elements:

Start where the patient is

Base assessments on an underlying view of what actually does happen to women in the world. Enable the woman to have a say in what goes on. Maintain and develop a dialogue to ensure that what is happening is understood.

Adopt an empowering focus

If advice or treatment is to be given (e.g. medication) it must be justified and make sense within the woman's life.

Real events need real action, e.g. housing, welfare rights.

Staff should be honest with themselves and the woman about the limitations to what they can achieve.

The commitment this type of work can involve for the worker can be considerable and must be acknowledged:

'I believe that some mental hospital patients may be casualties from being too often let down by people who could not contain them, resulting in an assumption that they cannot safely express the intensity of their feelings to any other person. And if someone ever dares such a patient once again to hope, that person can expect to be tested repeatedly for the anticipated failure and rejection .... With some damaged patients we take on a terrible responsibility. We could make things worse for them if we fail to survive at the point when they most need to test our capacity for survival. So we should only offer con-

tainment in a relationship, as an alternative to medication
or to hospital containment, with a full awareness of the
risks that may be involved. We must know what we could
be taking on.' (Casement, 1985: 145)

Mental health workers most likely to be involved with women
who have been severely damaged by experiences which they have
not been enabled to work through, are often likely to be working in
a hospital or day care setting. They will not and should not have sole
responsibility for such women. The most basic requirement is for
such women to be treated with respect and consistency and within
careful boundaries. The onus is on all those working with them:
nurses, social workers, psychologists and doctors, to work together
to ensure that the relationships established with the women involved
do not reproduce previous painful experiences.

Women such as Betty, Janet and Nancy may well have had early
experiences of abuse, rejection, loss or fragility related to the
important caring figures in their lives. Their later relationships may
well have echoed these earlier dynamics and their relationships with
the professional staff responsible for their care will inevitably
contain the same elements. Staff need knowledge and training to
understand this as well as a skill base to enable them to work
effectively. Equally important is careful supervision that can help
to ensure that the needs being met are for the abused and rejected
women to be heard, not the staff's needs to control the chaos they
represent.

Previous abusive relationships should not be re-enacted. It is
important, for example, to recognise that women can be used and
abused physically and sexually in hospital as well as in the outside
world. For example, a woman whose only valued role in the past
has been to clean and care for others may well be tempted to such a
role again if the new setting allows for it! Rather than encouraging
a woman to continue to measure her value in this way, it is important
that staff work with her to think of other ways in which she can be
valued appropriately.

For those who have not been so fundamentally damaged but have
had severe mental health problems throughout their adult lives,
poverty, instability in their accommodation, and a high degree of
social isolation are likely to be just as significant as their 'diagnosis'

in determining what help social workers and others need to be able to give. Practical help and the creation of a network of supportive relationships may be as significant as therapy in helping women regain control of their lives. A woman of 60 now living in a group home, but who had previously had admissions to hospital describes her relationship with two women with whom she now lives and who she had met whilst in hospital:

> 'We used to go and have a chat with each other and probably walk down to the town together, or go on the bus . . . well I got to know Elsie first, we was like friends, you know, we got on as friends and then Betty came, . . . and then they used to come for us to go and do cooking and that, on our own, . . . to see how we coped all together . . . well they could see as we could do it like, so when we came here we more or less went everywhere together . . . we help each other, I mean you help, that's the way life goes isn't it it, that's life, helping each other . . . if one goes out, another one goes with her . . . we went into town, went visiting, in the park, went to the pictures.' (Quoted in Ritchie *et al.* 1988.)

Summary

The important elements of loss and change in mid-life may well confront women at this stage with unresolved aspects from their earlier lives that still merit being heard, even if it is their small girl's voice from 40 years before. The tendency for this to be ignored in our anger at our mothers is clear. In some respects the case illustrations above exemplify the 'invisibility' of women in mid-life as well as the fact that available services, even that of grief counselling, seem only provided in terms of women's roles as wives and carers. It is as if society remains crassly determined to make mother see our need for her still to perform her duties to us before she can be deserving of our care.

A non-sexist approach would recognise women in mid-life have needs in their own right as they deal with the transition into old age and attempt to help them aim towards greater creativity and self-satisfaction, perhaps in less traditional ways, seeing this as an opportunity to develop aspects of themselves not needed previously. A community that was able to value the experience, wisdom, organisational and management skills of the average middle-aged woman would also be able to look at her greying hair and wrinkling skin without requiring her to hide them and herself!

5. LATER LIFE – OLD AGE:
Queen Mother or Old Hag?

'When I talk about old women at conferences and workshops, I invariably hear some of the following remarks:
I'm not old; I don't feel old; I don't look old; You don't
look old; don't call me old; why do you call yourself old;
you don't look 64; 64 is not old; Why do you use that
word? Old is a dirty word; old is an ugly word.' (Siegel,
1990: 90.)

Images of old women may be benign — the Queen Mother,
bizarrely feminine — Barbara Cartland, or frightening — the Old
Crone. They exist in a fairy tale world and are unencumbered with
positive power in any way. Any old woman who deviates arouses
our anger, at her threat to control us or the fact that she is not
providing the care of us we expect. We need to go to other cultures
to find a role model of a competent, wise old woman — Mother
Theresa of Calcutta for instance.

The vast majority of people over 65 in Britain are active,
reasonably healthy and mentally alert: only 2% of those over 65 live
in residential accommodation and another 2% live in hospital
(Crawley, 1988: 7). Yet society tends to think of them, if it does at
all, with reluctance, as recipients of care, as prospective makers of
demands on our busy schedules and already-over-committed
resources, rather than as people able to contribute to the community
in useful and responsible ways. Sheila Green, a 38-year-old nursing
student, disguised herself as an 80-year-old pensioner and was
abused and treated as an irritant when shopping, travelling on buses
and in a hospital out-patients department. She described her
treatment (Daily Telegraph, 18.8.91) as making her feel isolated, at
times frightened and most of all angry. Without the disguise but
with the same behaviour, she was treated with humour and
friendliness.

Attention to the political aspects of ageing has only recently
begun to receive interest from social policy and social work analysts
(see Bowl, 1986) and, as we noted in the previous chapter, even

feminists have been tardy in focusing their interest on older women. Those who work with elderly people are not exempt from ageist prejudices (Finch and Groves, 1985). We quoted Shere Hite in the previous chapter on the ambivalent feelings women have about their mothers. Siegel also writes of this:

> 'The ambivalent mother-transference that is directed at middle-aged women becomes more frequent and more pronounced as women get older. Ageism, the fear of aging and the fear of death now combine with unresolved feelings towards mothers and mother figures to confront the old woman with painful rejections, avoidances and invisibilities.' (Siegel, 1990: 91.)

These are feelings which those working with elderly women are likely to share and which must be confronted if practice is not to contribute to the oppression elderly clients may experience.

For many health professionals, functional problems in their elderly patients are seen as merely a natural and irreversible part of aging and organic deterioration: 'What else do you expect at your age?' is a typical comment and an observation which many old women have learnt to share. Hospitals still put older people at the bottom of the waiting list for non-urgent medical treatment and doctors generally view elderly patients as less exciting and less rewarding than younger people because there is no cure for old age (see Wilkin and Hughes, 1986).

Psychoanalysts originally believed people over 50 to be a poor investment for therapy, too resistant to change or simply untreatable and, whilst this view has modified as older people have manifestly challenged such ideas, ageist sentiments still abound in otherwise-creative workers in the 1980s:

> 'Budman. . . . has begun to experiment in short-term group work with all ages with a focus on life stage issues. In Later Midlife groups he had a different structure from the other age groups, for there was a 'revolving door' format. Members could attend for up to 20 sessions a year, but never really terminated, for after resolving their acute problem or crisis they left with the understanding that they

could return whenever they felt the need. This was because Budman considered that in a short-term therapy group for Later Midlife members, the experience of feelings regarding termination might be too stressful and anxiety-provoking.' (Hunter,1985, 49.)

Too often, old people are viewed by the rest of society as both sexless and genderless, but Sheila Peace's reminder that gender remains a key factor in people's experience of life as they grow older is an important one. Wilkin and Hughes (1986) suggest that there is evidence that people's health in old age is more a product of their experiences throughout their lives than of old age *per se*. We suggest that this is no less true for mental health than for physical health.

The increasing proportion of women in the mental health system becomes overwhelming amongst the oldest age groups. The fact that more women than men survive into extreme old age is only part of the reason for this. Elderly women were over-represented amongst those referred to social workers for possible action under the Mental Health Act 1983: they were referred at a rate of 92.2 per 100,000 compared with 56.3 per 100,000 men (Barnes, Bowl and Fisher, 1990). In the same study it was found that 72% of those aged 75-84 who were referred were women and this figure increased to 80% of those aged 85 or over. Once again official Department of Health figures confirm this: in 1986 73% of those between 75 and 84 and 81% of those over 85 formally admitted to psychiatric hospitals were women.

People in their 70s, 80s and 90s in the 1990s were socialised into assumptions about appropriate roles for men and women in the first third of the twentieth century when choices for women about how to live their lives were even more constrained than they are today. Life expectancy has also increased and older women in the late twentieth century are likely to outlive their partners and to experience lengthy periods of their lives living alone after their partners have died and children have left to create their own families. Their role as primary companion, nurturer, housekeeper and lover no longer exists. In the typical family in contemporary western society the grandmother has, at best, an intermittent role of felt usefulness; whilst she may be called upon to undertake some babysitting duties, her expertise in child care may be challenged by current views. By contrast with her earlier role of caring for others, she herself may now become a source of anger, worry and conflict within her family when the issue of who is to care for her when she can no longer care for herself arises.

We know that elderly women are amongst the poorest people in the population and that their financial situation is highly dependent on their previous marital status (see Hunt, 1978; Townsend, 1979; Peace, 1986). Nor is this a purely British phenomenon. As Tish Sommers, the first president of the American Older Women's League, remarked:

> 'Motherhood and apple pie are sacred in our society, but neither guarantees security in old age' (quoted in Hooyman, 1987: 264).

The objective circumstances of elderly men and elderly women are often very different. Both circumstances and self-perceptions of elderly women need to be understood in the context of the role they have played as women throughout their lives as well as in relation to their current roles.

It is hard to find any consideration of gender differences or their implications in studies of the origins of mental disorder in old age. In a study which aimed to adapt that of Brown and Harris in order to explore whether social factors are causally important in depression in old age, Elaine Murphy matched her sample using gender as a variable, but did not use it as a variable in the analysis of the data, nor did she explicitly consider gender as a potentially significant factor in her discussion of the results (Murphy, 1982). Key factors identified in her study were that depression is

> 'closely associated with adversity; events involving loss or threat of loss were implicated, just as in younger people. (p.140).

Physical illness also appeared to be a significant factor because of the fear of approaching death. But what she described as a 'major vulnerability factor' was the personality of the individual, specifically the person's capacity for intimacy. Other studies (e.g. Garside, Kay and Roth, 1965) have also suggested that personality characteristics associated with sociability are related to the experience of mental disorder in old age and it is such characteristics rather than objective circumstances of living alone which are significant. These studies do not consider the possible relationships between gender and personality in this context.

A study which considered psychosocial adjustment amongst elderly women and men from different ethnic groups in the USA found that overall there was little difference amongst men and women. However, there were differences amongst the different ethnic groups (white, black and Cuban) and the level of self-esteem was lowest amongst the white group (Linn, Hunter and Perry, 1979). In another small scale study, elderly people living in residential accommodation were interviewed as part of an investigation into self-esteem in later life:

> ' . . . these people are looking back on life as survivors; most of the people they knew when young have died. Survival in itself brings an element of self-esteem with it . . . . We noticed that what from an objective viewpoint were absolutely appalling events did not necessarily tend to a subjectively low esteem. For instance, one lady had had to cope in childhood with the death of both her parents, had been brought up by aunts and had then spent the rest of her life living in other people's houses, as a maid and untrained nanny; apparently a lonely life, without security or any long-term relationships, apart from with one of the children she had looked after who had since kept in touch with her. She looked back on this life, however, with serenity and contentment, saying that she had been lucky to have so much to do with children.'(Smith & Newman, 1982.)

The relationship between self-esteem and life experiences will depend on women's abilities to make sense of those experiences and to maintain a sense of their own identity and needs throughout. Linn *et al* (op.cit.) suggests that the attention given to women's rights issues in the media may have improved women's concepts of themselves. If that suggestion has any foundation in truth then it provides an optimistic indication of the way forward towards increasing the self-esteem of elderly women. Does self-esteem have anything to do with personality? At a common-sense level it seems reasonable to suggest that if your self-esteem is low then it is difficult to be sociable and to achieve positive relationships with others. Throughout this book we have described how a woman's self-perception and self-esteem can be challenged and undermined by the stereotypes which both confine her and present her with an impossible image to live up to. It does not appear to us surprising that elderly women whose personal and financial circumstances are often less secure than older men's and whose lives have been lived with a perception of themselves as in a supporting role to those who no longer need them or who may no longer be there, should more often experience mental distress.

The additional problem of chronic disability or ill health is something that older women more often experience than elderly men and Garside *et al.* (1965) have demonstrated a very high correlation between 'a general illness factor' and psychiatric illness. Gray and Isaacs (1979) suggest that neurotic reactions can result from stresses such as loss of employment, status, relatives or health and that a combination of social and psychological approaches designed to improve self-esteem are needed. Personality as a factor influencing an elderly person's feelings of loss, uselessness, loneliness and anger with a world that no longer makes sense to them is not something that can be understood separately from that person's experience of life. And that experience itself has been lived as a woman or man with all the differences we have been discussing throughout previous sections of this book.

Much of the research concerned with the provision of social work and social and health care services for elderly people is service-rather than needs-focused. The gender composition of users is often noted as a fact, but rarely is gender a variable which provides a basis for analysis. For example, one study which aimed to give prominence to users' views in the evaluation of a service was Evans's *et al* study of a travelling day hospital for elderly mentally ill people. (Evans, Kendall, Lovelock and Powell, 1986.) Of the 35 users of this service interviewed by the researchers, 27 were elderly women. The potential significance of this was not commented upon, nor was there any exploration of any differences in responses to the service according to gender. The researchers did consider the different marital status and household composition of the men and women users of the service and noted:

> 'There are differences between living alone, living with a spouse who is probably elderly him or herself and possibly therefore physically or mentally too frail to give much care or support, and living with a younger relative. The needs of the elderly mentally ill patients themselves, and of their varied family carers where evident, are all of concern to the TDH: the service aimed to offer support and relief to family carers, and to provide social contact and a focus outside the home for those living alone' (Evans *et al.*, 1986: 96–97).

However, apart from noticing that there was a difference in the living circumstances of the women and men there is no consideration of whether the service acknowledges those gender differences in determining appropriate ways of working with the users and providing support to their carers.

Finch and Groves (1985), however, discuss how apparent gender blindness in responding to the needs of elderly social services clients in fact reveals gender stereotyping at work in the provision of services. They draw attention to the higher number of elderly women who are defined as being mentally ill and suggest that this is only partly a function of the higher numbers of elderly women in the population. They suggest that toleration of certain types of behaviour, particularly aggression, will be lower if the behaviour is exhibited by elderly women rather than men or younger people. The higher referral rate of elderly women for assessment under the Mental Health Act (see above) tends to confirm this.

Annette Warner, who spent a week as a participant observer in an old people's home, gained a high level of insight into the experiences of the residents, most of whom were women. She described one woman's reaction to being admitted:

> ' . . . an elderly lady, who was very shy, felt she had been 'pushed into' the home by her daughter who wanted her

house, and so felt very rejected and frightened by the prospect of moving to a home. Her response was to shut herself away whenever possible and be unpleasant to everyone so they wouldn't disturb her.' (Warner, 1987: 16.)

It is not hard to imagine how her behaviour might come to be defined as evidence of mental disorder.

A clear demonstration of the relevance of gender is given at the start of Barbara Gray and Bernard Isaacs book 'Care of the Elderly Mentally Infirm'. They describe two contrasting case studies of elderly people whose mental state is providing cause for concern to others. One is an 87-year-old woman, the other a 65-year-old man. Their analysis is not a feminist one, but the circumstances they describe have much to say about the different life experiences of men and women and how that affects the response made to them. In Mrs. W.'s case the doctor was called by neighbours because she was walking in the middle of the road clad only in a tattered open dressing gown. Mr. S.'s brothers and sons called in the doctor when he started making what they considered unrealistic decisions about the family business which were likely to affect its profitability. Key characteristics of the two circumstances were as follows:

Mrs. W.

— She was much older and had been behaving in a 'strange' way for some time.

— She lived on her own most of the time and would not allow friends, health or social services workers in the house.

— Help was provided on different days by her son and his three daughters. The son was living on sickness benefit and his daughters all had jobs, children and husbands to look after as well as keeping an eye on Mrs. W.

— The description of her concentrated on her physical appearance. There was no description of how she had lived her life, other than that she had coped well, even though her memory was becoming impaired, until the death of her husband.

— Referral was caused by behaviour which shocked the neighbours.

Mr. S

— He was much younger and, although having reached official retirement age, was still working as chairman and managing director of his own company.

— We are told nothing about his physical appearance.

— We are told about his history in terms which suggest how individual endeavour had overcome an unpromising start.

— His 'odd' behaviour related to his work.

— The referral was made in order to certify him as medically unfit to prevent an adverse effect on the business.

In the previous section we suggested that the invisibility of middle-aged women was an important factor in considering their experience of mental distress. These examples suggest how that might carry on into old age. Because Mrs. W.'s life is lived in the private rather than the public sphere, her needs can be left to family to take care of, however difficult that might be for them. Only when her behaviour spills out and becomes public does she get a response. The signs that there is something wrong are that she is neglecting her physical care, and losing inhibitions about appropriate dress and behaviour. In Mr. S.'s case the 'symptoms' relate to his behaviour in the economic sphere and because this is regarded as very important there is a swift response designed to prevent harm being done. Gray and Isaacs point out that in neither case was the medical intervention helpful as both people died soon after.

Confusion in Old Age

Amongst elderly people, as amongst younger people, mental disorder can have a variety of forms. Gray and Isaacs (op.cit.) provide a useful explanation of the varieties of mental disorder in old age which draws on both psychiatric and social understandings.

The stereotypical mental disorder and that which is perhaps most feared amongst older people and their relatives is that labelled dementia. The term 'dementia' implies a range of symptoms which include memory deterioration — usually the first indication, disorientation in time and place, emotionality, loss of drive and lowering of inhibitions and standards of behaviour. The condition is caused by organic deterioration in the brain. There can be a variety of diagnostic labels: Senile dementia, multi-infarct or arteriosclerotic dementia and Alzheimer's disease are the most common, but it is important to be aware that other conditions such as head injuries, tumours and certain metabolic disorders can also cause similar symptoms. Therefore a careful medical examination is always essential.

There is, as yet, no clear understanding of the origins of the organic deterioration which results in dementia nor any successful treatment for what is usually a chronic and progressive condition. Prevalence amongst the elderly population is estimated to range from 1 in 10 of the over 65s, to 1 in 5 of the over 80s and as such dementia with its overtly identifiable manifestations is the most apparent mental disorder of elderly people in the public perception. Also associated with the early symptoms can be depression and anxiety as the old person is often aware at this stage of what is happening to them:

Flora

Flora was 67 when she first noticed that her memory was becoming erratic. A widow for the past 10 years, Flora was living alone, save for the company of her dog Jenny, for the first time in her life. Her two adult children were settled with their own families and busy lives, and although her daughter would visit every Sunday, Flora found that time could hang quite heavily during the week, especially when bad weather prevented her taking the long walks she enjoyed with Jenny.

Flora tried to fill her time. She took up keep fit classes and advertised for a lodger for her spare room and, at first, she could laugh off her memory lapses. She would suddenly forget the name of a common object she was trying to describe and sometimes she would put a saucepan on the stove, only to forget she had done so and to find it had boiled dry when, for instance, she returned from a long walk with the dog. Gradually, however, these incidents became increasingly more common and more worrying, both for Flora and her daughter. The day came when Flora was found in distress at the former family home, now occupied by another family. Flora had thought she still lived there and could not understand where her husband and young children were. Sadly, Flora was now always to be 'wandering', trying to find her way to the home that no longer existed. Her children arranged for her to move to a nursing home where she could be looked after and prevented from wandering away. Here she was given medication for her anxiety and her distress seemed to alleviate. Her children suffered the pain of watching their mother deteriorate to someone who no longer recognised them nor perhaps mercifully understood her situation until her death a few months later.

Dementia is slightly more commonly diagnosed in women than men. Can a feminist understanding have anything useful to say in relation to this type of mental distress in old age? We believe so. It may not be appropriate to search for causes in the particular life experiences of women — although one could hypothesise that the greater stimulation of the brain through the working life of a man could be preventive, just as any other muscle in the body can be maintained to a high standard of fitness by regular use. But the way in which the condition is experienced and the response which may be offered *are* likely to be influenced by gender.

Those working with severely confused women and with their carers need to develop a practice which acknowledges the part that gender has to play in the changed relationships which result from the changes in personality and behaviour associated with what we know as dementia. One implication of this as far as elderly women themselves are concerned relates to the identification and prioritisation of work in health and social care agencies. Once again there is a danger that the needs of women may remain invisible for longer because they are contained within the private life of families. As far as practice is concerned, it may be important to rediscover the woman's history, not to ignore this as of no significance. Current reality is often fragmented and confusing and the tendency is for people suffering in this way is to be treated in a paternalistic, even dismissive manner. It is almost as if to suggest that with the loss of their mental and physical acuity and independence, people suffering from dementia have also lost the right to respect. One way to make real contact is by helping the sufferer to remember and explore past experiences. The major emotional relationships and events in a life nearing its end have already taken place and part of the psychological 'work' of all our old ages is to make sense of and accept what has happened to us. Recall and reminiscence tapes are being used with many groups of older people. These involve sharing pictures and sounds from common earlier life experiences such as the two world wars and the depression in the 1930s. Workers using the currently available tapes comment on how these are able to arouse even highly confused people to speak lucidly about their past but the tapes which are widely used contain predominantly male images. Workers committed to the use of reminiscence therapy would do well to produce material which provides positive images of women's lives.

Reality orientation therapy is another method used to help elderly confused people remain in touch as far as is possible. Here, usually in a residential setting, workers constantly remind residents of the important facts of their current lives, e.g. the date and time. These efforts are backed up by an environment equally conducive in terms of well-lit, easy-to-read clocks and calendars supported with clearly available and reiterated information about other aspects of day-to-day life. This system has been found helpful in delaying further deterioration and tends to support the view, already discussed, that social and emotional isolation in old age contributes towards deteriorating mental health conditions.

Other workers use different creative ways of communicating. Art therapists describe innovative methods of enlisting the interest of older people to a form of expression often last used 60 or 70 years ago. One worker spoke of introducing her group to mandalas, the Eastern symbol used for meditation. She explained the purpose of the symbol and its shape, intricate but uniform, and suggested people used colours that pleased them to illustrate their picture of the mandala. The worker was rewarded by a quiet and spontaneous absorption as what were normally very distracted people were able to work rhythmically, creatively and with unusual concentration.

Meditation and healing; physical therapies such as massage — which can also address the lack of oxygen to the brain of people sitting in one position for too long; Tai Chi — a measured form of controlled, gentle exercise; the Alexander Technique — a form of re-education of the body posture which involves a gentle moving of the body by the therapist; these are but a few of the methods of working with older people with mental health problems which utilise the link between psyche and soma for communication and improved self-confidence. Some of these would seem particularly appropriate for work with groups or individual older women in enabling those who feel fragmented and isolated to feel held, communicated with and cared for in an acceptable way.

Carers

Being confronted with taking on the care of an elderly relative, partner or friend raises uncomfortable issues for most women. Caring for an elderly person experiencing mental distress can make extreme demands on patience and tolerance. Work with carers will sometimes have to include helping them to deal with the loss of a relationship even whilst the person is still alive.

It is perhaps this element of loss which, coupled with what one Alzheimer's Disease sufferer's carer called a '36 hour day', can lead to 'granny bashing'. Many carers, some of whom are as elderly if not older than the person they are caring for, describe feeling pushed to the limits of their patience and tolerance by the experience of living with a confused woman who may, for example, ask the same question several times within minutes only to forget the answer immediately. Living with someone who seems careless or even aggressive about their personal hygiene, or whose anger seems irrational can arouse in the female carer anger and frustration she feels it inappropriate to express. It may also stir up ambivalent feelings, such as those about mothers we have already identified. Holding these feelings in can lead to a point where an often physically and mentally exhausted carer can respond aggressively herself. Often the carer will be a male spouse who may need help in coming to terms with a caring role which is not only something of which he has no experience, but which he might find threatening, puzzling and extremely distressing. Gilleard (1985) reports a study which found that male carers found it easier than women to receive help from professionals to support them in their caring roles. The author of this study suggested this was because men did not identify themselves so strongly with the caring role. But some men may find it difficult to identify with other carers, most of whom are women, and therefore not be able to benefit from the support offered by carers groups. One of us has found this in work with a group of carers set up to monitor developments in services for carers. A male member of the group spoke of feeling excluded from what he saw as a woman's world. The reversal of traditional gender roles, particularly for elderly people whose expectations were formed before these were being challenged as publicly as they are today, may be hard for both carer and cared for.

Depression and anxiety in old age

Elderly women are often described as 'confused' when their thoughts or behaviour seem illogical to the observer or they are disorientated in place or time. This 'confusion' can be an early indication of dementia or depression but it may equally well be caused by other factors. There may, for example, be a variety of physical causes, from a high temperature and fever, through to impacted faeces; or even practical issues such as a lost hearing aid or glasses. The apparent confusion may also be an accurate reflection of reality. It is important not to jump to conclusions!

'One old lady was almost taken to a psychiatric ward, because she was found hammering on the door of a shop an hour before opening time — it turned out that her clock (her son's responsibility) was one hour fast. No one had given her the chance to give her version of what was happening. Another lady was diagnosed as paraphrenic, because she complained of being followed about and abused by a gang. Her social worker accompanied her on a shopping expedition (keeping at a distance) and, sure enough, a group of boys marched after her, calling her names like 'witch' and worse!' (Hudson, 1982: 93.)

She may also be suffering from a recent trauma or life event that may be considered a normal occurrence in old age without our acknowledging the distress involved. For example, a move from home to hospital, or from home to stay with a daughter can be experienced as an additional stress by an older woman who may also be trying to deal with the emotions surrounding other losses and changes in her life.

The high rate of depression in old age often goes unrecognised or is wrongly diagnosed as dementia. A range of depressive conditions can occur, from severe depression with a risk of suicide through to appropriately reactive depression as the old person experiences the many life changes and losses that occur in old age.

Recognition of the depression is the first step to an intervention aimed at reducing the distress. Thus it is important for families and professionals alike to bear in mind that they might know not just a lonely old woman, but a lonely, old and unhappy woman. However, much of the difficulty in communicating appropriately with the old woman's feelings is because it involves facing our own ageism, our own fears of growing old and dying. When we busy ourselves with practical tasks, by attending sometimes over assiduously to the physical needs of the older woman, when we attempt to 'jolly' her 'out of herself', we may do so from our own resistance to being in touch with both her and our own emotions that can include a mixture of pain, guilt, anger and distress.

Mavis

Mavis's father died when he was 87 and she was 65. She was left alone in the family home where she had lived with her parents since her younger brother left home in his 20s. Her history was a sad one. Her mother had apparently devoted her life to looking after Mavis who never washed herself, her own clothes nor learned to cook or clean. She did , however, manage to hold down a job for some time in a shop and was also married at one stage, although the marriage quickly broke down and Mavis returned to her family from the caravan in which she had set up home. Some years later, she also had an illegitimate baby but because it was considered that Mavis would not be able to look after him, her son was adopted soon after the birth and Mavis never saw him again.

When first her mother, then her father, died Mavis's brother and the neighbours blamed her for working them so hard to look after her. She was considered lazy, selfish and only interested in herself and a steady supply of cigarettes. She also had a variety of diagnoses that she had acquired over the years — schizophrenia, borderline personality disorder, possibly mentally handicapped , none of which had been successful in achieving a treatment plan that would bring about long term improvements in her coping abilities.

On her father's death, the local social services department attempted to assess her abilities. Since she didn't cook and clean for herself at all, the available domiciliary services were organised. She was found to be able to respond to basic behavioural task setting and management but her anxiety at her isolation at home on her own for the first time ever was unbearably painful. Mavis was given a trial in a rehabilitation hostel but was eventually considered unsuitable as she showed no wish to learn to care for herself. She would enlist her fellow residents in looking after her needs. She was subsequently found a place in a residential establishment for the elderly where her dependency needs are met and her anger and distress at her life experiences, her present surroundings and their lack of stimulation are managed by tranquillising medication.

In essence, Mavis could be considered to have been failed by her devoted parents who despite their best intentions, allowed her to become institutionalised at home, neither able to become appropriately interdependent nor to develop a life of her own. Nor did the professionals involved in her care through the years act pro-actively on Mavis's behalf. It could be concluded that the paternalistic attitude which affected her parents' view of her colluded with Mavis's own anxiety and fear of separation. Her response to the eventual losses, both current and past, seemed only possible to be contained and managed by medication rather than allowed the necessary expression as a first step towards releasing the energy she needed to claim a life for herself.

We believe there was a gender issue here. Did it appear to the family that Mavis needed the protection from herself to prevent further sexual adventures, in much the same way that many young unmarried mothers were deemed by their relatives as in need of the care and protection of the large mental hospitals and are only now, as elderly women, coming back into the community as these close? Also, would a man who had not been taught to take responsibility for his own care receive more sympathy than did Mavis? Mavis's story demonstrates the dilemmas deriving from a view of dependence as pathological when such dependence may have been encouraged as appropriate for a young woman. Seligman described the syndrome of 'learned helplessness' which occurs when the individual feels she has no power to control the environment upon which she is dependent for survival and suggests that elderly people are often treated in ways likely to lead to such a state (Seligman, 1975). The residential establishment to which Mavis moved, a privately run organisation, made sure that they provided a high quality of physical care for their elderly residents. Unfortunately, little stimulation was provided for their mental well-being with the staff constantly busy attending to physical needs. Concentration on meeting the physical needs of elderly people at the expense of their emotional well-being reinforces the dependence we pathologise.

There are many organisations devoted to improving the health and welfare of groups of older people in our society. Both Age Concern and Help the Aged, for example, function widely on both practical and policy levels enlisting community support through volunteer workers and fund raising, to provide a range of services which include luncheon clubs, social events, home visiting and counselling of both older people and their relatives. Other projects focus on differing aspects of older people's needs; for example, the Beth Johnson Self Health Care Project in North Staffordshire seeks to raise awareness amongst older people of health issues generally, including important aspects such as diet, exercise and relaxation patterns. They also provide a telephone call service, where old people considered to be at risk are contacted on a regular basis in order to monitor their health and bring some communication from the outside world to someone otherwise confined and isolated.

We view these services as invaluable, filling as they do the gaps where statutory services are not available and in some instances providing an alternative model of service. Local authorities and hospitals also provide a range of residential and day care services for elderly people in their areas within which dedicated workers attempt to meet some of the needs we have discussed above. But few of these services directly address the mental distress elderly women may be experiencing.

Managers and workers need to recognise the institutional defensiveness in services which often aim to meet the physical needs of their elderly users whilst disregarding their equally important mental health needs.

Resources and services to older people all too often are provided by volunteers and unqualified workers in a low priority service when compared, for instance, with the priority reserved for child care in social services departments. Our ageism certainly shows through here as does the fact that we still find few settings where older people are invited readily into groups of users of mixed ages.

Loss, dying and death

Patricia

Patricia was born into what she describes as a 'well-to-do' home, the youngest of three children. Her father commited suicide when she was four and her mother remarried shortly after, to a man who beat Patricia. She describes herself as a bit of a rebel who married early to a 'working class man'. 'Perhaps I was looking for a father, or I just wanted to get away from home.'

The marriage was far from a success, as Patricia had no idea how to cook and keep house, so it was something of a relief (possibly for both of them) when her husband was called up for armed service in the war. Towards the end of the war, with her husband still away, Patricia met John. She was pregnant when she heard her husband was coming home. She could hear the V2 rockets falling on London as she gave birth to her daughter and thinks it was the guilt and confusion that contributed to the post-natal depression she experienced. She tried to jump out of the hospital window and worried about being only maimed rather than dead.

Patricia's life since then has been one spent as a 'mental patient'. She was diagnosed 'manic-depressive' and alternated between periods at home with John and their three children and time spent in long-stay wards in hospital. Some of her experiences there she describes as brutalising. She has made further attempts on her life and she believes the stress of this contributed to John's becoming an alcoholic. Fourteen years ago, however, she was put on lithium, a mood stabilising drug, and since that time her life has been much more equable.

Her children have now left home and John has died. Patricia, however, described herself as having 'triumphed', with her husband's continuing love and support as well as the lithium, and believes that through all her struggles she had an inner core of resilience that determined her survival.

One of us met Patricia at a mental health drop-in centre that she uses on a regular basis. Now living alone, Patricia finds the company and support she needs in this resource which provides an essential lifeline now that her family are no longer so available to her.

As they approach the end of their lives, older women are confronted with the inevitable losses that accompany this time. Most must learn to face increasing isolation as partners and close friends die, children develop their own preoccupations, and physical infirmities if not financial restrictions limit travel and social activity. As we have discussed, this is a time when depression and anxiety can be expected and, as with women such as Patricia, other longer-standing problems remain to be managed but now without the support of partners and family.

In recent years, those involved with working with older people in different environments, in their homes and in the community and residential settings, have begun to look at more innovative methods of improving communication, between professionals and clients as well as amongst the older people themselves, mainly through the use of group work in various forms. Whilst we have found very little specifically aimed at the needs of older women, some of the techniques being used with mixed groups could well translate.

Older women as well as younger women can benefit from sharing experiences which cause depression. Joan Hunter describes an incident in a group she ran for elderly people:

> 'Enid was the only one in her group who was not con-
> fused. She had only recently moved into the residence
> where the group was being held, and was in great distress

because her sister, with whom she had lived all her life, had died. In the first session, she was frantic and kept calling out 'Betty', the name of her deceased sister. In the second session she shouted, 'I wonder why I have to live at all? Why shouldn't I be allowed to do us all in?' I repeated to the group that Enid was asking why she has to go on living. I added that we don't know — you have to wait till your turn comes. Rachel at once said, 'It's just as well we don't know.' At about this time, Lena said, 'Conversation keeps you together. When we are together we get to know each other. When you recognise a person you talk to them'.

It was interesting that Enid, in spite of what she had said seemed to have experienced being accepted by the group. In the next session, she began to change, she joined in talk about what was good to eat and asked another member if she felt quite well. She also said, 'You can't stop time — it just goes on,' as if she herself had accepted what she could not control.(Hunter, 1989: 13.) Here the worker was able to talk about death undefensively and by so doing, seems to have enabled Enid and the other group members to feel that even their more uncomfortable and seemingly anti-social thoughts and feelings could be accepted and shared without fear of rejection. Hunter describes her pleasure and surprise when, visiting a group a year after finishing her regular contact with them, she found that members remembered her, despite being considered generally confused and absent-minded, and also remembered the atmosphere and culture the group had provided.

Groupwork provides specific therapeutic factors which are particularly relevant at a stage in life where isolation is common. Foulkes, a psychoanalyst who developed group analysis, described them as follows:

> (1) The patient is brought out of his isolation into a social situation in which he can feel adequate . . . .
> (2) The patient's realization that other people have similar morbid ideas, anxieties or impulses, acts as a potent therapeutic agent, in particular relieving anxiety and guilt . . . .

116

(1) The patient is brought out of his isolation into a social situation in which he can feel adequate . . . .

(2) The patient's realization that other people have similar morbid ideas, anxieties or impulses, acts as a potent therapeutic agent, in particular relieving anxiety and guilt . . . .

(3) Many more themes are touched upon and it is easier to talk about them when they have been brought up by others . . . .

(4) Explanations and information . . . are of course not peculiar to the group situation, but in one respect there is a significant difference: that is the element of exchange.'(Foulkes, 1964: 33.):

Groupwork can be an empowering and collaborative model which has much to recommend it when working with elderly women. Foulkes' ideas of group analytic psychotherapy have been mainly developed in long term, open-ended mixed gender groups of seven to eight members with a leader called the group conductor and with little structuring of group interactions, other than that the group should attempt to share their problems. Time-limited models of groupwork are also useful for members with a particular common interest, e.g. recent retirement, bereavement issues, as these models allow for the common theme to be explored but with a view to this focus being identified as a transitory stage from which people will eventually move on. As with all groups and, indeed, counselling and therapeutic work with individuals, workers would find it important to discuss with a supervisor or consultant issues such as preferred models, client selection, group process and leadership, if the group is to achieve optimal success and effectiveness.

We are reminded, of course, that the growth of feminist ideas has developed traditionally from the experiences and shared understandings of women meeting together in groups. Feminist groupwork practice can, in our view, be a forum in which to address many of the personal and political issues for women's mental health that we have been discussing in this book. By sharing their feelings and experiences in groups, women can begin to understand some of the structural factors affecting their lives that they may wish to

We believe that for most women sharing in single gender groups can offer the social validation necessary for improved self-esteem and confidence and we would thus generally recommend the development of work with such groups of women clients as a high priority for the feminist mental health practitioner. There may be times when a more heterogeneous group make up is appropriate for particular women clients, but this will usually be subsequent to time in a single gender group. Anyone planning to work with women in such a way may well wish to refer to Butler and Wintram's book, 'Feminist Groupwork' (Butler & Wintram, 1991), whilst for ideas for self-help therapy groups for women and group exercises, we recommend Ernst and Goodison's 'In Our Own Hands' (Ernst & Goodison, 1981).

Dying and death itself are another stereotype which needs to be confronted if the positive aspects of the older woman's life are to be identified. Elisabeth Kubler-Ross (Kubler-Ross, 1969), whose work has transformed the care of the dying, speaks of five stages of dying: denial, anger and bargaining followed by an opening up to the depression and sadness of loss which allows the move on to acceptance.

Levine (1986) quotes a woman given a terminal prognosis who, after struggling with the confusion of the early stages, found herself 'opening to the uncontrollability of things'. She experienced a new freedom, a spaciousness she had never known. She said that even more important than *death* becoming more acceptable, *life* had become acceptable. A few months into that openness she had a complete remission. She suspected that it was her opening to death that allowed life to come back into balance. She said, however, that as she looked back at those years when she was considered terminal,

'I was never so alive as when I was dying'. (Levine, 1986: 241.)

Thus our old age, a time when we look both backwards over our lives and forwards to a greater unknown, offers an opportunity to live our lives in the present more fully than ever before. Levine's view of dying proposes that there are opportunities of old age rather than merely negatives. Whether we have a deep religious faith or not we can,by bearing to explore it,convert our view of death froming a frightening enemy, an end of everything, into a transformation, an opening, a rebirth.

Once death no longer seems so destructive, all of us, old and young, can be freed to live more fully. As women, we may be uniquely well placed to take the opportunity of enhancing our mental health in this way, to use our abilities to be open to relatedness, to feelings, to share and communicate them in old age as perhaps never before.

An example of what we are trying to describe here is that of the mother of someone known to one of us. In her old age, she began talking to her daughter and telling her of her feelings about her for 'if I don't tell you now, I never will'. Mothers and daughters sharing in old age can heal the old ambivalent relationship, spiritually and psychologically; an experience that can contribute to the mental health of both women, as the following words from a woman after her mother's death describes:

> 'I just forgave her, and I forgave myself for some of the hatred I had had toward her. I was really beginning to reckon with her as a person; who had real feelings, who had been hurt and stunted and blighted in some fashion. I could separate myself from her at times enough to simply see her as that human being' (Robbins, quoted in Siegel, 1990,: 50).

Social workers with elderly clients and those who work with women who are caring for their elderly mothers need to understand how this exploration of ambivalent feelings might be necessary both as a direct approach to working through mental health problems, and if the daughter wishes to continue to provide personal care. Without enabling such an exploration to take place, unresolved feelings could well make the role reversal involved in daughters caring for their mothers impossible to achieve both at an emotional and at a practical level.

Summary

'I use the word old deliberately, in order to reclaim it. Having learned from Black women and men that black is beautiful, I would apply that lesson to old, using the word to desensitise us from the fearsome connotations of old. If we are to love our aging bodies, we can start by changing the language and begin to see that old is beautiful.' (Siegel, 1990 op.cit.: 90)

The number of very old people in the population is going to increase, whilst the numbers of young elderly (65-74) will diminish. We must beware of presenting that fact in a way which implies that the old people are causing us a problem by their survival. What it means is that we must learn better how to respond to those whose old age does not bring peace and contentment, but increasing mental distress resulting from life experiences or organic changes. Women, presently in their 60s, 70s and 80s were brought up with limited expectations and their distress may be easy to ignore. Fears of being labelled 'geriatric' and sent to what they perceive as the workhouse may also have prevented them from seeking help. The next generation of older women will include the feminists of the 1960s and 1970s. Many of those involved in service provision are realising, with Clare Ungerson, that 'Policy is Personal' (Ungerson, 1987) and yet have to come to terms with their own ambivalent feelings about their mothers before they can develop a practice and policy which does not continue to reinforce oppression.

For older women to claim their mental health we need to share with them, to understand their oppression which results from our sexist and ageist prejudices and structures. Men, women and children need to acknowledge our fantasies of power and nurturing, rage at and then accept our own inadequacies rather than allocate them to our chosen scapegoats. Only then can older women be appropriately empowered as well as cared for, be dependent and independent and rightly find appropriate interdependence in a society that can benefit from their skills rather than deny or grudge them the respect they deserve.

6. WOMEN AND MENTAL HEALTH LEGISLATION:
Mad or Bad?

There are times when women's mental health problems become both severe and public in a way that results in consideration of the use of the controlling powers of mental health legislation. The existence of such legislation is evidence of the right claimed by society to act against an individual's wishes if those professionals (doctors and approved social workers) to whom power is delegated consider that this is 'in the interests of his own health or safety or with a view to the protection of other persons'. (Part II Section 2 (2) (b) Mental Health Act 1983.) They must also have decided that the person concerned is suffering from mental disorder (Section 2), or 'mental illness, severe mental impairment, psychopathic disorder or mental impairment' (Section 3 of the Act) and that such a condition is sufficiently severe to warrant assessment and/or treatment in hospital.

The characteristics of such legislation and the implications for the decision making of social workers with responsibilities for putting it into practice are discussed in some detail in Barnes, Bowl and Fisher (1990) and in Sheppard (1990). From the perspective of the individual woman on the receiving end of compulsory powers the following quotation sums up the position:

> 'At base, the Mental Health Act defines what may be called mental disorder in our society, and under what circumstances the freedom to seek or disregard treatment may be suspended and the individual obliged to accept medical advice. To be sectioned, therefore, means to have no choice in how some piece of behaviour is to be interpreted and called evidence of mental disorder, no choice in whether to seek help and accept treatment — these decisions, and the sense of personal autonomy that they engender, are taken out of your hands.' (Barnes, Bowl and Fisher, 1990: 12.)

Anyone can refer someone for assessment for compulsory admission to hospital. Only those whom the law designates can take the decision to admit. Information about the characteristics of people referred can give some idea of both professional and lay assumptions about the circumstances in which people should be 'taken away for their own good'. Information about who is actually admitted gives a particularly professional view of this.

We know from Department of Health statistics that over half of compulsory admissions to hospital are of women. We also know that the proportion of women compared with men changes with age. Under the age of 35 more men than women are admitted, but once over this age the balance changes and the proportion of women increases with every age band.

Information about who is considered for compulsory admission is not officially collected in the same way. For some indication of the decisions which are made about referrals and the outcomes of these we have to look to the small amount of research which has been conducted in this area. Once again the question of gender is rarely seen as an issue to be explored in decisions whether or not to invoke the power of the Mental Health Act. Race is more often seen to be something which should be considered (e.g. Rogers and Faulkner, 1987; Ineichen *et al.* 1984; Szmuckler *et al.* 1981).

The apparently unproblematic nature of gender in this context, as in other considerations of mental health practice, makes the task of arguing for the development of anti-sexist practice more difficult. Hospital managers when asked by one of us why they thought more women than men were admitted compulsorily into their hospital appeared completely nonplussed. It was not a question that they had before been asked or had asked themselves. Even in a recent study of ASW decision making which had an explicit aim of developing practice which is based on social science knowledge, the relevance of gender as a factor which could influence decision making was not explored (Sheppard, 1990). But our previous discussions about both the experience of mental disorder and the response which women receive suggest that it is unlikely that gender is a neutral factor in the application of legislation when it is not in other areas of professional practice. The analysis to which one of us contributed in a previous project confirms this (Barnes, Bowl and Fisher, 1990).

This study of referrals to social workers for action under the mental health legislation explored the characteristics of those who were referred, and compared outcomes for people in different circumstances. In both instances gender appeared to be a significant factor. Not only were women referred at a higher rate and slightly more likely to be compulsorily detained following an ASW assessment, in those cases where admission did not take place and alternative care was provided there were observable differences in the alternative sources of support used. Family support was seen to be available and/or appropriate in 47% of cases where the woman was not admitted, but in 39% of cases involving men. Residential care was rarely used generally, but it was used least when the alternative care being sought was for a woman between the ages of 35 and 64. We suggested one reason which may underlie this:

> 'Entering hospital can be legitimated by 'being ill' and 'needing treatment'. It will involve temporary disruption to family life and arrangements may need to be made for the care of children whilst mother is away. In extreme cases this may involve a temporary reception into care. But moving to other accommodation, which cannot be seen as a place where a cure for an illness can be found, is more challenging. If the family is seen as the fount of succour and the place where its members seek nurturing, why does one of its members who is not sick need to move elsewhere for support?' (Barnes, Bowl and Fisher, 1990: 136.)

It may be argued that residential resources simply do not exist for men or women in that age group. That in itself is evidence of the extent to which it is assumed that people in distress will be cared for at home within the family environment. The problem for women is that they are more often than not the ones who are providing the emotional support.

One woman who spoke to us, Marjorie, described her role in life as 'the middle person', the bridge builder, one who would listen and arbitrate between conflicts both at home and at work. The assumption that at times of distress women such as Marjorie will themselves be able to call on the necessary support may be mistaken. If family relationships have developed over the years on the basis of one person filling the supporting role it simply may not be possible for role reversals to take place when they are needed.

We know from conversations we have had with women who have been cast firmly into the caring role how difficult they have found it to both seek and receive emotional support from their families when they have needed this.

Before considering what responses might assist women whose mental health problems have reached the stage at which some public response is demanded, what do we know about the characteristics of those circumstances? The majority of the situations described below are drawn from a random sample of 100 monitoring forms completed by ASWs during the course of the Mental Health Act monitoring project.

Situations in which the woman is considered to be a danger to herself.

This is implied by the reference to compulsory admission in the interests of the safety of the person concerned. The actual circumstances in which a threat to the safety of the woman is considered to exist are extremely varied: they can apply to women of all ages; to women who are already hospital in-patients as well as those for whom hospital admission is being considered; such danger can be seen to derive from both deliberate self-harm or neglect and from the implied behaviour of others as well as directly resulting from the woman's own action or inaction:

> Girl (23) had come from lodgings in London in an agitated state. Threatening to harm herself, said she'd lost her identity and needed help. Frightened and upset, refusing (initially) any medication.

> Very agitated and depressed. Danger to self if allowed to leave (hospital). Tried to throw self out of window prior to admission. Not eating, sleeping. (59-year-old.)

> Client suffers from chronic anorexia nervosa (last 15 years). Has no insight, refuses to take adequate nourishment. Present weight only 5 stone 12 lb. Risk to life exists if not sectioned and client refuses informal status. (58-year-old)

Voluntary patient. Then refused to eat or accept medication. Dehydrated and likely to die. Client depressed, suspicious and unaware of the seriousness of her depression. (74-year-old)

A rather different type of danger was pointed to in this example from Sheppard's study of ASW decision making:

> In the past she had been at risk of going out late and chatting up men. It hasn't happened so far, but on past performance I expect it would.

It is hard to imagine that such a justification for the use of compulsory detention would be provided if the client were male.

One very strong impression which is left by these and other descriptions of women considered to be endangering themselves is of the chronic lack of self-esteem which they feel. At a recent conference on the subject of self-harm and at which personal presentations based on experience were made, it was acknowledged that whilst self-harm was not confined to women 'the majority are women and many of the apparent triggers to self-harm seem to be connected to women's particular position in society — sexual abuse and 'food distress' for example' (Campbell, 1990: 7).

This impression is reinforced by glimpses of the closed environments of the special hospitals. Many of the women who are in these hospitals are there because of their actual or perceived danger to others, but their experiences of life and of being detained in a total institution have caused many of them to engage in self-mutilation of a quite horrific kind. Research carried out by staff at Ashworth Hospital has identified that over 88% of women detained there have experienced sexual abuse at some stage in their life. Prue Stephenson in an article in Openmind provides one of the few descriptions of the experiences of women in these environments (Stephenson, 1989):

> 'Sylvia, currently in Moss Side . . . was physically and sexually assaulted from an early age. She could not settle at school, ran away from home on several occasions and spent most of her time alone . . . In 1984, when she was

18, she was arrested and convicted of assault and was sentenced to two years in prison. Most of her sentence was spent on the psychiatric unit in Holloway (C1). At that time, due to staff shortages, women on the unit were frequently locked up 23 hours out of 24. Unable to read and write (a life-line for many women in prison), Sylvia spent many hours alone in her cell. During this time she self-mutilated, damaged her cell, showed violence towards staff and set fire to her bedding . . . .'

Whatever the origin of behaviour which demonstrates neglect or more active attempts to harm herself, a woman who has reached this stage is likely to need a therapeutic response which focuses specifically on her own self image and how she can build her self-esteem. Admission to hospital may be necessary to provide security, asylum and, in some instances, treatment, but this alone is unlikely to provide the basis on which such rebuilding can take place.

Situations in which the woman is considered to be a danger to others.

Those with a diagnosis of mental disorder, mental illness, psychopathic disorder or mental impairment can be admitted to hospital against their will if their behaviour is such that it is considered that other people need to be protected from it. One of the factors which the Department of Health's Code of Practice on the Act suggests should be taken into account in assessing for this possibility is 'the willingness and ability to cope with the risk, by those with whom the patient lives' (Department of Health, 1990). The importance of how others perceive behaviour and the extent to which they are able and willing to tolerate it are thus made explicit. The fact that people exhibiting similar behaviour in very similar circumstances may thus be treated differently is not made explicit.

Women are more often than men in situations in which they are providing care for others who may be dependent on them. The stress that such a role can produce, whether from caring for a small child, for an adult son or daughter with severe learning difficulties or for an elderly parent who may be frail, incontinent and confused, can be an underlying cause of mental distress. The ability of the person being cared for to cope with the risk from behaviour which may result from such distress is likely to be low. Thus women may be more often considered to present a risk to others because of the nature of the relationship they have to those others.

We have discussed how aggressive or deviant behaviour amongst adolescent girls evokes a stronger response than similar behaviour on the part of boys. Violent and aggressive behaviour generally is regarded as abnormal in women; it can produce a shocked reaction amongst professionals as well as amongst friends, family, acquaintances and strangers. Such behaviour can be regarded as evidence in its own right of madness.

The first example quoted below describes a woman who could harm herself as well as others. However, it does illustrate quite well how the response of other people is an explicit factor which affects the way in which women are treated, as well as how concern for (in this case unborn) children will influence decision making:

> Patient's behaviour impulsive and unpredictable — bizarre and quite unacceptable to all around her. Unable to hold rational conversation (Pregnant 30/40) Caused fire in kitchen. Stepped into moving vehicle. Generally a danger to self and others.

> Had visited the local Bridewell the night before claiming various strange things. She absconded from the station before section forms could be completed. The family reported her at home the next day. She was verbally violent and at one time attacked her daughter. She intimated that she was being interfered with. There followed other bizarre acts.

This woman had a diagnosis of paranoid schizophrenia. With such a label it may be that her suggestions that her daughter is being 'interfered with' are automatically regarded as a symptom of her illness. Evidence that her concerns are simply regarded as confirmation of her madness could add to her despair and, indeed, her daughter's isolation.

Harm to others can be seen to derive from neglect as well as active behaviour:

> 36-year-old living with husband and children. Client suffering from religious obsession and neglecting family. Reported to be ill. This woman was not admitted to hospital.

Less obvious direct harm is implied in some of the circumstances leading to referral for assessment, but a mother's behaviour towards her children is a key reason for the referral being made:

> Single mother with a history of manic depressive illness. Preventing her child from going to school as she was paranoid about infection being around.

In the following instance the woman was not admitted to hospital. The woman had been diagnosed as suffering from schizophrenia, but the social worker called to assess her observed: 'No sign of mental illness, matrimonial dispute' —

> Client at police station following complaint of ABH by husband. Wife said to have hit him with pick axe handle during manic outburst previous night. (40-year-old living with husband and children.)

Once again it is possible to imagine the likely differences in the action which would have been taken if it had been the husband attacking his wife. Referral for assessment for compulsory detention in a psychiatric hospital may not have been a likely response.

Crises involving family and relationship difficulties.

Women who have been interviewed about the origin of their mental health difficulties can often identify very clearly what for them have been the factors leading to their distress. Sylvia Bailey talked to users of a mental health centre, the majority of whom were women. Amongst the factors they identified were: financial problems, marital problems, death of a close relative, lack of social outlets and isolation, problems with children and physical health problems. She described one woman's experience:

'She had supported her daughter through divorce, had worried about her husband's excessive drinking, had helped her father after his cardiac arrest, helped her mother after his subsequent death, all combined with a demanding job and a chronic illness. In addition the dog had died and three other relatives. So much for her strength! She commented that she found it hard to get angry (a comment often made by women).' (Bailey, 1987: 31.)

Such knowledge is often denied by medical practitioners who understand disordered behaviour in terms of the symptomatology of illness. The relationship between life events and mental distress is not a straightforward one, but for the practitioner who is concerned to help women attain a way of life which contributes to their mental health, helping women to understand why such events have led to difficulties and how to develop strategies which can avoid future problems should be at the centre of their practice.

Crisis intervention approaches are based on

'the premise that when people experience life changes, whether accidental or developmental, they experience disruption in their psychological 'steady state'. When they are unable to cope with these changes they may enter a 'crisis state' with associated feelings of intense anxiety, depression, agitation and so on. If help is provided to resolve the crisis in a positive way individuals may re-cover their previous psychological 'steady state' or even an improved level of functioning. However, a maladaptive response to the crisis may result in poorer levels of functioning and mental health'. (Cantley, 1990: 1.)

Few of the social services departments involved in the study of Mental Health Act referrals had a crisis intervention service they could draw on. The need for such a service was identified in 21% of 'preventable admissions' taking place during office hours and 26% of 'preventable admissions' taking place out of normal office hours. (A preventable admission was one in which the ASW concerned considered that hospital admission could have been avoided had alternative sources of care been available.)

Descriptions of the circumstances leading to the assessment referrals indicate the type of 'accidental or developmental' life changes which have particular meaning for women and which led to them being considered for compulsory detention:

A girl (17) with a disturbed family history — Care. Recently her baby was placed on a care order. Following voluntary admission to psychiatric hospital she discharged herself to her mothers home and showed aggressive, bizarre, psychotic type symptoms and panic behaviour.

Patient 'high' and aggressive. Unable to cope with 2-week-old baby. No insight.

Patient felt desperate through lack of sleep. 6 weeks ago lost a baby — full term, died shortly after. Husband in Nigeria working, needs him and more support.

Widowed 4 months ago. Depressed and has taken to drink. Psychiatrist concerned she may be a suicide risk. (38-year-old)

Tense weekend at home. Fiancè here, planning August wedding. Monday evening fiancè returned home. A. very depressed, attempted suicide by trying to jump out of the window. She kept talking of death, wanting to die, had various other methods in mind. Total refusal re hospital admission. (25-year-old living at home with her parents.)

In each of these circumstances the immediate crisis in which both the woman herself, and potentially other people, may be at risk needs a response which will contribute to and not detract from longer term work. There are circumstances in which the bizarre and difficult-to-understand behaviour which can result from mental distress leads to stresses and breakdowns within family and other relationships. The woman is then left with both the problematic behaviour which precipitated the breakdown, and the fact of the breakdown itself. In other instances, whilst there may be no absolute breakdown, the strain of caring can become too much and outside help is desperately needed. Referral for consideration of compulsory detention may be the only way to guarantee some response from professional agencies, but will that response address the impact of the fractured relationships which have occurred?

> (78-year-old woman with senile dementia.) Husband who had been supporting his wife left her on Sunday. Son had stayed with her since but unable to remain to look after her. Client confused and unable to look after herself, no awareness of danger, wandering also, no insight into illness, refusing voluntary admission.

> This woman had not spoken a word for 18 months and her husband finally decided to seek help. She had suffered from delusions in the past. She had taken to her bed when I visited but refused to speak to myself or the consultant.

> Patient showing signs of paranoia. Some signs of thought disorder. Verbally abusive and aggressive to all. Refusing all treatment/help. Some refusal to talk to professionals, but not consistently. Husband emotionally worn out by her consistent bombardment of him. (60-year-old woman living with husband and children.)

In all these cases and in others where the description is of bizarre, frightening, dangerous or aggressive behaviour, resolution of the immediate crisis is not enough. Fear of a recurrence of such an experience, the knowledge that decisions have been taken out of your hands, that existing relationships may have been threatened or destroyed and the underlying questioning of self-identity that crises of mental disorder can bring, all mean that the women concerned are likely to need continuing support, practical assistance and therapy.

The reality is often very different. In only 36 out of the 100 cases sampled for the above analysis did the social worker undertaking the assessment stay involved with the woman after the assessment had been completed. This is virtually the same proportion (35.2%) as applied in the study as a whole. Some concern about this was expressed in an earlier report of the project:

> 'What this points to is the persistence of a tendency for the majority of clients to receive a short-term, one-off service, followed by referral elsewhere in about half the cases of compulsory admission and no further action in just over a quarter. Recalling earlier evidence that about a quarter of people referred had previously been known to social services, the obvious question arises as to whether these are the same people. In other words, does social services have its own revolving door?'. (Barnes *et al*, 1986: 42.)

This idea was supported by a small scale study (Maple, 1984) of social work practice in a London borough where during the study period (two months) Mrs. D. was referred twice in crisis:

> 'She has a diagnosis of schizophrenia and, although still living on the premises of a business theoretically jointly managed by her husband, is now the subject of divorce proceedings. The result of both referrals was that she was referred on to the psychiatric services following a duty social work assessment. Once a community psychiatric nurse was asked to call and once Mrs. D. was admitted. No social work intervention aimed towards the psy-cho/social and practical problems surrounding the fami-lial breakdown took place at the time of either crisis. With (such) stressful living circumstances . . . it is hard to see

how the pattern of such referral will not be repeated indefinitely.' (Maple, 1984: 46.)

'Evidence from both the United Kingdom and the United States suggests that social work with people in emergency situations in which the use of legislation is being considered is not popular. Where work is interpreted as coercive because therapy has failed or is simply not available, it forces social workers to be aware of their 'social policing' roles at the expense of their roles in assisting self-determination or the attainment of rights' (Satyamurti, 1979; Emerson and Pollner, 1975). However, Fisher, Newton and Sainsbury's in-depth study of mental health social work in one authority suggested that the opportunities available to social workers assessing people with a mental disorder were perceived to be much more constrained than in the case of the equally coercive task of receiving children into care:

> 'Workers seemed often to adopt the simplistic view that, where a client was mentally disordered, any risk-taking behaviour must necessarily be the product of mental disorder and must be prevented at all costs. This uncritical attitude towards risk, and the assumption that hospitalisa tion was a safe course, underlay the process of assessment, and stood in marked contrast towards social workers' attitudes towards the assessment of children at risk.' (Fisher, Newton and Sainsbury, 1984: 171.)

Sheppard's work (Sheppard, 1990) reinforces the view that ASWs are applying for compulsory detention solely on the grounds of the mental disorder of the person concerned and that potential danger to health or safety is viewed solely as an aspect of mental illness itself.

The contrast between responses in cases of mental disorder and responses where care of children is the focus of attention is undoubtedly a result of the relative priority given to those types of work in social services departments and to the resultant differences in the amount and range of resources and interventions open to them. But this is not the whole story. Whilst the 1983 Mental Health Act designates the Approved Social Worker as the only professional who can actually make the application for compulsory detention, social workers are frequently perceived, and perceive themselves, as being in a subordinate position to doctors in anything to do with mental health.

In Fisher, Newton and Sainsbury's study they found an unofficial policy amongst social workers in the authority that if a referral for an assessment for compulsory detention came from anyone other than a psychiatrist, then a psychiatrist's opinion should be obtained before the social worker visited in case such a visit was unnecessary. This study took place before the passage of the 1983 Act and one of the intentions of that Act can be seen as the promotion of the role and responsibilities of social workers in the implementation of the legislation. However, it will take much more than the implementation of new legislation to redress the balance in the relative powers of medical and social work professionals in this context.

ASW training in its early days was confused in both organisation and purpose. Much of it was dominated by the acquisition of medical and legal knowledge and the sociological and psychological knowledge base on which social work practice should be built received much less attention. Whilst knowledge was tested in the examination, social work practice skills were not. (For a discussion of this see Barnes, Bowl and Fisher, 1990: 121–126.) Within social service departments the new approved social workers could not be sure that their supervisors or managers had as much knowledge of mental health issues as they did, nor that they would get support for follow up work with individual clients let alone any development work they might want to pursue (Barnes and Prior, 1984).

In this context what possibilities are there for positive work with women experiencing severe mental health problems and who are being considered for compulsory detention?

Responses

The Chinese symbol for crisis means both danger and opportunity. The Concise Oxford Dictionary defines asylum, in the original sense that the Victorian philanthropists used when developing the large hospitals we still know today, as a refuge, a sanctuary from external stress and demands. We suggest it is appropriate to look at both these ideas when attempting to develop a non-sexist response to women in emotional crisis.

Sara Hutchings, a user of the mental health services, speaks of her experience of being compulsorily admitted:

> 'My fear of psychiatric hospital was such that I felt I would lose my freedom, my autonomy, and my already delicate sense of self, all in one go. I was also terrified that going into hospital would confirm my worst fear — that I was mad or bad or both.... What confronted me when I arrived was a group of nurses and doctors who, with the policemen, immediately surrounded me, pushed and pulled me into a side room where I was held down on a bed and injected — it felt more like being stabbed — with a substance which I later found out was Largactil.
>
> ... that ... instilled a further mistrust in me of psychiatry and the kind of help it can offer. It made me aware of the profession's enormous powers and shaped my belief that a variety of other services are needed for people in crisis. As a woman, I also feel that if other women could have been brought into the situation when I was in crisis, the air of physical confrontation could have been reduced'.(Hutchings, 1989.)

Hutchings' experience seems far from 'sanctuary' and much more like a punishment for unacceptable behaviour! What is needed she believes:

> 'is a trained person with the appropriate skills to enable the distressed individual to regain their confidence and control over their lives. Such a relationship on a one to one basis for a short period of time, preferably in a warm caring environment (a crisis centre), might be a decisive step on the road to recovery.' (ibid.)

Crisis intervention centres offering overnight accommodation such as she mentions are few but her description fits the crisis intervention service run by Coventry Social Services Department.

This operates from a large house in a residential area of the city, is staffed by male and female social workers and nurses and offers a 24 hour service aimed at immediately responding to people presenting in crisis, either self-referred or referred by other mental health professionals. This service, favourably reviewed by Cantley (op.cit), aims at qualities of normalisation, positive response, equality and confrontation in their involvement and users particularly appreciated that the team members had time to address their problems in depth, had specialist expertise and often could offer continuity of contact. The majority of users of this service are recognised as having 'neurotic' rather than 'psychotic' problems and the team see this specialism as adding to their effectiveness as opposed to that of other community mental health agencies who attempt to deal with a wider range of emotional distress. Sadly, as we write this chapter, we learn that continuing funding for this service is currently being reconsidered.

Women's centres of various kinds have developed in different forms and address some of the needs of women in distress. Women's Action for Mental Health in West London is an agency that offers mutual support to women in crisis in a neighbourhood setting and sees their strength as deriving from their self-help nature. Shanti, a women's counselling service in South London, provides a drop-in service staffed by women of different cultures, and Lambeth Women in Mind have set up a telephone counselling service for women. However, we are not aware of similar projects with residential provision. We believe that the extent of the crisis needs of women in emotional distress is still barely recognised, as these and similar resources in other parts of London are so marginal to the mainstream of mental health services and, in Shanti's case too, in imminent danger for lack of funds.

Crisis intervention workers are aware of an opportunity to be influential with people in crisis if the service is provided at the time of distress, before a maladaptive solution is found and some form of equilibrium, whether it be a return to the *status quo* or not, restored. A crisis intervention service for women, staffed by women, on the lines of the Coventry team might be an ideal to be aimed for. Given the chance, such a service might also be able to widen its scope to look at women suffering from what are termed psychotic reactions as they relate to feelings of grief, loss, anger, anxiety and despair at the social discrimination they experience. Obviously there will always be a need for some women in distress to have access to short, and even medium, term residential facilities offering the sanctuary of a breathing space away from the reality of their lives. However, we also believe that crisis intervention strategies can be adopted by workers attempting to respond to women in crisis, whether or not there is a formal crisis intervention service available. We suggest that asylum can mean psychological space where comfort and understanding are accessible, and need not always be seen as a physical space.

Felicity

Felicity was 20 when she was referred to the hospital self-harm unit from the casualty department where she had gone when she felt no longer able to cope — neither with a physical condition, for which she needed medication and should have seen her GP, nor with her college work, or with overwhelming feelings of helplessness and despair. The unit to which she was referred is a specialised consultation unit within the hospital which concentrates on work with people presenting with ideas of harming themselves, of overwhelming distress and various emotional problems. It is staffed by both medical and counselling staff.

The social worker in this unit helped Felicity initially to identify the issues that were contributing to her stress. Her father had died two years previously and she had never grieved for him. Her mother, who had been violent and abusive to her, and her disabled sister lived some distance away and Felicity felt responsible for them but also very ambivalent. Not sure whether she deserved to be a student, she was setting herself incredibly high standards for her course work and was working sometimes around the clock to achieve them. She also had financial difficulties which she was partly attempting to deal with by working in the evenings as a care assistant and, for relief from work, she would go to the gym to work out. In all, Felicity was exhausted, both physically and mentally.

At first, Felicity saw the fact that she needed help at all to be a huge weakness. Like many people who have coped with needy feelings in a family where showing vulnerability risks abuse, she had managed by controlling herself and her feelings, as if she feared that letting them out could risk overwhelming chaos. Having resolved the initial practical problems, she needed to think over the social worker's suggestion of brief therapy. The temptation was to return to a pattern of coming for help only when she was in crisis.

Subsequently, she decided to go ahead with therapy and a contract for work together was agreed. Initially, the sessions were difficult — Felicity would either maintain her isolation by missing sessions, or she would overwhelm herself and the worker with endless facts. Here too she demonstrated her dilemma:

Either absolute control (of self, life, others, work) or overwhelming chaos (both inside and out).

By structuring the therapy and focusing on this way of Felicity's functioning, the two women were gradually able to make sense of their experience together and Felicity began, tentatively at first, to share her feelings with the worker in a genuine way. She began to understand that many of her problems had originated from her fear of her mother and her childhood belief that the only way to be acceptable to her father was to be his 'little boy'. She spoke movingly of her fears of not really belonging in the academic world she had found herself in — a far cry, it also seemed, from her working class origins and, as she shared these ideas, she gradually became able to take more risks. She became more creative in her work and even let herself have some social life. Aiming now, to allow more mutuality into her relationships, as therapy ended, Felicity shared her feelings about the loss. She allowed her therapist to know how important she had become for her, both in words and by sharing with her some of her, by now, truly high-standard-work.

We believe that this short piece of therapeutic intervention with a woman in considerable distress is a useful model for other mental health workers to consider. In her relationship with the worker, Felicity found care and understanding for herself, not for what she could offer as in her other relationships. She became able to share her vulnerable side without being abused or humiliated. In essence, the therapy relationship was the sanctuary, 'the asylum', that enabled Felicity to build her self-esteem sufficiently strongly to develop a more constructive way of functioning than she had previously. The modifying of her fear of intimacy and loss of control should also allow her much more satisfactory relationships in the future.

Women who present in crisis are likely to have histories that include early deprivation, loss or separation, or other rejection by important figures in their lives. Having experienced this, they are sometimes overwhelmingly needy and reject themselves. They tend to elicit ambivalent behaviour from the professionals they meet. A clear structure for crisis intervention work, with a contract for the number of meetings and the focus of the work, should be a protection for both worker and client against misunderstanding, premature ending or disappointment at the limitations of the work. Felicity and her social worker spent some early sessions dealing with the practical issues that needed to be resolved first before making their contract to focus on relationship issues.

The model of intervention used with Felicity is similar to that described earlier which was used by Carol and Josie's social workers. Since it pro-actively involves the woman receiving therapy in collecting information and participating in the experience in an active way, we believe it is an empowering and helpful way of working with women in crisis in settings as varied as general practice, hospitals, alcohol rehabilitation agencies, forensic psychiatry, drop-in centres and other voluntary projects.

Summary

Women experiencing mental health crises are more at risk of being compulsorily detained in psychiatric hospitals and wards than are men. This fact, like other gender differences in mental health statistics, is treated as largely unproblematic by those running the services. Resources to prevent admission to hospital are in short supply generally, but there is evidence that family support rather than non-family help is used more often as a preventive resource with women than it is with men.

Paradoxically, women who are considered to be in need of psychiatric hospital admission are more likely to be living in families than are men and stresses which are part of family life have been identified by the women concerned as significant causes of their distress. Also, the role of women as carers within families may mean that they are more likely to be in a position where behaviour resulting from mental disorder could be regarded as actually or potentially dangerous to others.

Bizarre or aggressive behaviour may be tolerated less in women than in men because it challenges stereotypical views of appropriate behaviour. The impact of such behaviour on relationships between the woman and important people in her life may further undermine the chronic low esteem which is a common experience of women with severe mental health difficulties. Those working with women in this situation will need to help them rebuild their lives both emotionally and practically.

Crisis intervention services can provide alternatives to hospital admission for many women. Crisis intervention could be practised even where formally designated services do not exist and workers could provide psychological asylum where physical space has not been set aside for this. A time-limited approach to intervention when women are experiencing severe difficulties could be both more sensitive to the real needs of the women concerned, and more 'efficient' in preventing repeated referrals leading to repeated psychiatric admissions.

7. FEMINIST PRACTICE IN CONTEXT

'There will be a power struggle because life involves such
struggles, and the hegemony of those doing well in it is
too lightly called common sense, while those angry and
smarting are called mad.' (Alec Jenner, 1988.)

Responsibility for implementing the type of gender sensitive
practice we are advocating cannot rest with individual practitioners
alone. A readiness for change in individual practice must be
accompanied by the creation of organisational environments which
support that practice. These must in turn be enabled by policies
reinforcing the significance of gender as a variable, which should
inform the development both of services and of practice. As we have
indicated at different points throughout this book, this is far from
being the case at present. Gender is invisible in much mainstream
research and policy making. This does not mean that policies and
practice are neutral as far as gender is concerned. In a world where
sexist ideologies which reinforce male power dominate, gender
blindness means that women's needs are often simply not
recognised, or worse, derided.

Feminist practice must develop within the context of progressive
mental health practice generally. That in itself must be based on an
understanding of mental distress which draws on social and
psychological knowledge and on the subjective knowledge of those
for whom mental distress is a part of their lives, as well as on the
psychiatric understandings which currently dominate mental health
practice. This view has implications for the professional power of
the psychiatrist in particular, as well as the power of other
professionals working within the mental health system.
Contemporary movements of users of mental health services present
a general challenge to the assumption that professionals necessarily
know best. Many of the arguments of those involved in such
movements about the need to develop new types of relationships
between providers and users of services, have much in common with
feminist analysis of the need for changed relationships both within
the workplace and between providers and the predominantly women
users of welfare services.

At the individual level that must affect the nature of the practice which is engaged in; at the organisational level it means opening up decision making processes to influences from outside the usual power structure. In some areas that opening up is taking place (*see for example* Croft and Beresford, 1990; Connelly, 1990; Barnes and Wistow, 1991), but there is a long way to go before these movements come to represent a fundamental shift in the balance of power between professionals and users of services. In the area of mental health in which the 'illness' model is pre-eminent, for women to assert that they have an insight into their difficulties which the doctors to whom they go for treatment do not have is to undermine the science on which the work is based. Alec Jenner, a psychiatrist who we quoted at the beginning of this chapter, whilst defending science, has acknowledged the political and ideological influence on what is accepted as scientific fact. He seeks shared decision making and a partnership between users and professionals to create the kind of environment in which mental distress will be minimised:

> Despite being aware of my own desire to win some affection from the User Movement, I must urge them to look at society's difficulties with those its structures and families may well have almost irremediably damaged. Certainly we can fight together for situations in which that will be less prevalent, as we should to have excellent nurseries, kindergartens and schools, so that all will feel wanted and inadequate parents will be less able to damage. We can also struggle for a multiplicity of houses, flats, hostels, employment possibilities and other facilities which will hopefully make interventions therapeutic and not damaging. Equally we must agree to look honestly at pharmacology and genetics and neither worship them nor turn a blind eye. (Jenner, 1988)

Much of our analysis throughout this book has suggested that early intervention aimed at addressing underlying causes of mental distress would have been beneficial to the women whose stories we have discussed. Jennifer Newton has argued the case for prevention rather than cure in mental health (Newton, 1988). If prevention is possible, and Newton provides convincing evidence of how it is possible to identify those who are 'at risk' and develop interventions designed to minimise that risk becoming a reality, then there is a role for a considerable number of players in contributing to prevention. Her identification of the type of preventive interventions which would reduce the experience of severe mental distress (see pages 234-237 of her book) would have made life a much more positive experience for many of the women whose experiences we have described here. Such a concept, however, is regarded with great scepticism by many psychiatrists reluctant to give up their control of that area of human experience which has become labelled 'mental illness.' What is equally worrying in the contemporary situation is that a general attack on 'welfare' has resulted in a widespread acceptance of the general need for targeting of resources on those who are already in severe difficulties. Early therapeutic interventions are often only available to those who are able to buy them privately.

Most feminist analysts of policy and practice would agree with other exponents of radical welfare practice that such practice cannot be developed in isolation from activity on a wider front in politics and in trade unionism (see for example Dominelli and McLeod, 1989, and Banton et al., 1985). But such a recognition should not divert attention away from what it is possible to achieve within existing structures, nor from how such structures may be reproduced within existing worker/client relationships. There is no point in social workers being feminists in their women's groups but not in their relationships with their women clients or their women colleagues.

In this final chapter we shall consider what this may mean at the level of policy as well as for the content and organisation of mental health practice which can assist women in mental distress. We will consider this first at the level of practice which has been the main focus of this book.

Practice

Throughout this book, we have identified the overwhelming need for women in emotional distress to be heard. The personal and professional stress caused when mental health workers come into touch with another woman's distress needs to be acknowledged and addressed if effective help is to be offered. In one social services department, a woman worker with a family where a female child had been sexually abused was sufficiently self-aware to recognise she was becoming overwhelmed by the feelings she was carrying about the case. She asked for access to a specialist consultant to help her manage the case, the demands of which were affecting her ability to deal effectively with the rest of her work. This was seen by her managers as a sign of incompetency on the worker's part and led to a management appraisal of the whole of her work, and the possibility of disciplinary action was raised. In another authority, and in conjunction with a voluntary agency, two women approached their respective managers with a proposal for work with sexually abused young women which included a pre requisite for external specialist consultancy for themselves in order to handle the work effectively. This was agreed to and their work, described in Chapter 2, has since developed to the position where the two organisations now see the group help based on this pilot work as a high priority part of the service response to sexually abused young women in the area. We see these differing responses as highlighting the individual and organisational issues that need to be addressed and negotiated if a gender sensitive mental health practice is to be achieved successfully.

There is an inevitable tension created within any organisation responsible for attempting to manage situations which can appear as otherwise likely to threaten our social order with chaos or anarchy, whether the organisation be a family, a hospital or even a local authority social services department. Menzies (1961), in a well-respected paper, described the defensive strategies developed by the staff of a hospital ward in an attempt to achieve control and order. She suggested these structures were maintained in order to control the anxiety that actually communicating with the distress experienced by their patients would entail. Similarly, by attaching a diagnostic label which identifies the person for whom we provide a service as different from us we maintain the 'them and us' dimension. In this way we can protect ourselves by identifying the chaos as belonging elsewhere.

Such strategies to control the uncontrollable are colluded with by the predominantly male managers and female frontline staff. They are a way of managing the stress and anxiety raised in human beings faced with pain and distress which would otherwise threaten to overwhelm. Ernst (1989) describes another defensive strategy which she suggests is equally prevalent within organisations, where one post, section or group of staff can become endowed, likewise in fantasy, with maternal powers. Like a mother, this person or group is seen as being able to nurture, protect and heal in a powerful way, suggesting she/they can help people to be 'human' in the organisation. In reality people in this position are unlikely to have real power or ability to influence organisational strategy and functioning. Ernst's description was applied to the post of a groupwork consultant to a social services department. Her conclusion, having worked in such a position, is that if organisations are to function more successfully staff need to give up their gender stereotypical fantasies and to recognise and acknowledge our lack of ability to control everything. Both women and men need to claim their share and take on the responsibility of real power.

Confronting gender issues in mental health and mental health practice threatens the defensive structures and strategies which have been developed at various levels, including unconscious ones. If the powerful father or the male-oriented management team can no longer maintain self-esteem by identifying weakness as the sole province of women and children, or female staff, or mad or bad service users; if mother's power to nurture and protect us from the demands of the real world is only illusory; if sanity and madness are on a continuum, then the fear is raised that it can touch all of us. If emotional and physical abuse is really taking place in families like yours, perhaps it can happen, is happening, in mine . . . .

The worker who admitted anxiety and asked for help, we believe, stirred such fears in her managers in the same way that the Cleveland workers with sexually abused children, and more latterly workers investigating ritual abuse of children in other parts of the country, stirred fears in the public. One result was that gender biased systems of control were invoked to control what were perceived to be stereotypically hysterical female or female-identified workers. It was far safer for a defensive management team to identify the individual worker asking for help as bad, than to acknowledge the insufficiency of their structures and strategies for keeping chaos (of which sexual abuse is a very potent symbol) at bay.

The workers involved in the group for sexually abused young women were in a stronger position. It is much more difficult to identify a group as misguided than it is an individual. Secondly, their work was meticulously planned and argued, proceeded slowly and was discussed with their managers at each stage. Having achieved this influential support within their organisations they were also careful to enlist the views of external specialists, to enlist received wisdom in support of their arguments and to incorporate the new learning as they went. Finally, we believe a considerable contribution to the success was their overall good communication. As part of the evaluation process, for example, the workers arranged for group members to attend a review meeting with the managers concerned, to discuss the experience and their progress together. In this way, fears and fantasies on both sides were translated into a manageable and rewarding experience.

What can we learn from this if we are to be able to influence mental health practice on a larger scale? Speaking out often means challenging the stereotype of 'good little girl' and as such can evoke earlier conflicts both in ourselves and in those we confront. One woman-centred mental health project we contacted had felt misused and even abused when they were misrepresented by the media. The understandable response to this was to keep themselves to themselves and not to talk about their work outside the project again. However, we cannot ignore the fact that by keeping silent women collude with their oppression and leave other women in ignorance and isolation.

Workers wanting to improve their practice need to share thoughts and ideas, to check with each other, to speak with united voices rather than singly, to avoid running the risk of isolation and disillusion. Those sympathetic to the promotion of gender sensitivity in mental health practice need actively to seek greater knowledge and information, to increase their skills in practice and communication and to achieve greater influence in the organisations, both by seeking powerful allies as well as by claiming responsibility themselves. It will not be given willingly and women, in particular, must increasingly put themselves forward to claim positions of influence. As women we need to operate at all levels in organisations and within different types of functions if we are to ensure that women's mental health problems receive a more sympathetic and appropriate response by the mental health system. We need also to develop appropriate strategies to protect ourselves. Support networks for women workers and managers, both within and outside work settings, could be better developed. Assertion training and public presentation courses will be needed to allow women to present themselves more effectively.

Joy Dalton described some of the steps she and other women colleagues took when attempting to challenge the male oriented *status quo* in medicine. An important first step was to identify allies and a women's support group of like-minded female doctors was developed. Dalton explains:

> 'The group met for about three and a half years on a fortnightly basis and became very important to us in many ways, which other women who have been in women's groups will recognise. It firstly helped us support each other by acknowledging the value of our own experience as women in our work. In the medical profession our experience as women was often devalued and ignored.'
> (personal communication)

She describes two incidents where the support of the group enabled women workers to challenge the undervaluing of a woman's experience of child rearing in a job competition, and also to face the opposition and derision which arose when members of the group tried to raise an issue of sexual abuse of a patient by a member of staff.

Mental health workers generally can also learn from psychotherapy the importance of the therapist herself receiving therapy. Banton and her colleagues (Banton *et al.* 1985) have written of the importance of peer and group supervision for therapists engaging in radical therapy. They suggest that the degree of openness and trust which such supervision requires may not always be possible to achieve within the work setting and may have to be sought outside. Recognition of one's own collusion with sexism in our society and where our own competitiveness and 'mother blaming' tendencies can interfere with our work and relationships with other women is the first step to working more sensitively. Increased training and gender-sensitive supervision can help to develop our effectiveness.

The groupworkers described above were able to argue effectively for appropriate consultation. We believe other groups of staff could similarly claim training and consultation to address issues related to the effectiveness of their work if they described it in ways which are consistent with the objectives of their organisation.

Changes in ways of working must be carefully planned, argued assertively and evaluated appropriately because mistakes and inefficiencies will be looked for, to be used as reasons for reasserting the old order. Sadly, the stereotype that, for women to succeed, we must be better than men, may well have some validity as attempting to change stereotypical work practices will not be easy or comfortable. Parimala Moodley (Chapter 3) suggested that this had been a significant factor in the success of her approach. The fact that social workers are still able to be stereotyped as well-meaning do-gooders suggests they may collude with the myth of omnipotence (Maple,1988). A reluctance to be clear about the aims and goals of their interventions, thus preventing evaluation of efficacy, gives comfort to social work's critics. For successful change to more gender-sensitive-practice, all workers should pay attention to the detail of their work, basing it on well-founded theories tested in practice by themselves or others, whether it be Self-in-Relation theories, group analytic practice or other more behavioural models of intervention.

Sexual abuse is a current example where much careful work has been and is being done to identify the value of specific interventions as well as to evaluate their ongoing preventive value in terms of future demands on services. This is leading to greater organisational commitment to fund such initiatives. Other specific models of intervention which have been well researched and include built-in evaluation structures, such as the cognitive analytic therapy model, may also be ways forward.

Perhaps the best known of the voluntarily run agencies currently speaking out to promote women's mental health is the Women's Therapy Centre. In the 14 years of the centre's existence, it has become known both nationally and internationally for its work aimed at promoting a better understanding of women's psychology. Whilst the centre provides women with a wide range of free or low cost individual or group psychotherapy characterised by a clinical setting without authoritarian relations or drug treatments, it also recognised the need to have a strong educational focus. There is a high priority for staff to write their work up. Training courses for mental health professionals to inform their work with women clients are provided alongside workshops on particular themes, such as eating disorders, loss and bereavement, managing stress, and women at work, which enable women to meet their own particular needs as well as to learn new skills. We understand these services are constantly over-subscribed with approximately 10,000 women contacting the centre each year.

The Women's Therapy Centre is by now well established, although financially precarious, and its success has contributed both to raising the profile of women's mental health needs and to the development of women-centred services elsewhere. Similar centres now exist in Leeds and central Birmingham, although society's ambivalence is still symbolised by the fact that these, like most other projects we have discussed, have had to seek funding from outside mainstream service budgets.

Policy

Developing services which are designed to meet women's needs means getting the issue of women and mental health on the policy agenda. Whilst we do not propose that this is exclusively the responsibility of women professionals, we do think that more women are needed in policy-making positions if this is to become a reality. We also think that a substantial increase in knowledge about women's experiences of emotional distress and their experience of the health and social care agencies which are intended to help them is needed to assist the process. In the previous section we have suggested that this needs to influence the content of social work and other practice training. This is no less important in training available for managers and policy makers. Co-operation between those in different positions within the system is necessary to achieve change:

> To meet women's needs fully, it is critical to understand the link between the four roles of direct service, advocacy, research and policy. For example, if a female policymaker is advocating for a mental health policy within a city, she must rely on the researcher to provide her with data about women's mental health needs; she must rely on the direct service provider to give her information about the specific unmet needs of women within that city; and she must rely on the community advocate to provide 'outside' community pressure on city government while the female policymaker is advocating 'inside' city government. (Stringer and Welton, 1984: 46.)

The following example of a policy issue may serve to illustrate this. There is much talk at the moment about targeting the development of community mental health services so that those who are 'seriously mentally ill' are receiving help in the community. In diagnostic terms the 'seriously mentally ill' are often defined as those with a psychotic illness rather than affective or neurotic disorders —'the worried well' as they are sometimes rather dismissively referred to. There are very positive reasons for this. There is a genuine concern that the development of community-based services should not exclude those whose mental disorder is very severe and long lasting. The danger from a feminist perspective is that this ignores the differential rates of diagnosis of different types of disorder in men and women. There is a risk that the pain experienced by many women who are crushed by depression or isolated by extreme anxiety is dismissed as less important than the often publicly bizarre behaviour of people defined as psychotic. Some evidence of this may be found in the work of Brown and his colleagues in a more recent study of women experiencing depression (Brown *et al.*, 1987). The women were more likely to have seen a psychiatrist for treatment if they had demonstrated some form of personality disturbance or 'acting out behaviour' as well as their depression. Measuring the differences in the level of pain experienced and hence the priority that should be given to providing help cannot be achieved solely by reference to the diagnostic categories developed by psychiatry. We do not suggest that there is an easy answer to this. What we do say is that such assumptions about the prioritisation of services is in itself a product of an ideology which has failed many women who have looked to 'the mental health system' for help.

So can an awareness of women's mental health needs reach the policy agenda? The United Kingdom looks as if it lags behind the United States in this. There, in 1977 The President's Commission on Mental Health established a sub-panel specifically to look at the mental health of women. The report of this panel has been described as 'a blueprint for the development of mental health policy responsive to women's needs and has become an organizing platform for women's mental health policy advocates'. (Russo, 1984: 22.) There is no equivalent at national policy-making level in this country, but in some areas moves are being made.

The West Midlands Social Services Mental Health Services Forum has produced a statement of philosophy and principles which includes an equal opportunities statement that discusses mental health needs of black people and of women (ADSS West Midlands Region, 1989). Whilst such a statement of principle may have only a very indirect effect on practice, it is important that it exists in a document which has the support of all Directors of Social Services Departments in the West Midlands. It can be used as a basis on which to argue for more specific service developments.

In one health authority known to us a group of women have gone further than that in developing a strategy for women and mental health. Their experience provides an example of some of the struggles which may be experienced, but also suggests some of the directions in which it is possible to move from within statutory services. It is worthwhile looking at what they have been trying to achieve and what has happened to them in the process. We have been asked not to identify the area concerned.

Their reasons for wanting to develop a strategy specifically concerned with women's mental health needs reflect many of the arguments contained within this book. They felt that orthodox psychiatry's response to women with mental health problems was often not helpful. There was a lack of therapy which explicitly recognised women's experiences and access to community mental health facilities was difficult for many women. This was in spite of the existence of a broad policy statement referring to the needs of women and ethnic minorities. They did not regard themselves as a particularly radical group, but could not fail to recognise that most of the people they worked with were women and that they were not able to meet the needs of all the women in the area.

The woman who took the lead on the initiative was the only woman on the management team in her area. She was asked to work on developing a proposal and in order to do this issued an open invitation to women working in the area to join a group. The group that was convened consisted of medical and nursing professionals, social workers, psychologists, health visitors and women from voluntary agencies and the Community Health Council. It was decided to make it an all women group and one result of that was that few of those who joined the group were in senior or powerful positions in the hierarchy. Later a woman who worked in the planning section joined the group and her involvement was considered crucial — she was described as 'a powerhouse' by one of the women we spoke to. She knew the system and was able to make links with planning processes and decision making forums in the authority.

As well as drawing on the experience of the women workers who joined the group, open days to which both workers and women users of mental health services were invited were held. Few users came to these meetings, but they were considered a useful way of identifying some of the problems with traditional mental health services which women had experienced. Resources were not available to undertake a more systematic survey of users' experiences.

The group did not want their proposals to be marginalised. They wanted the services they were proposing to be a part of the overall development of community mental health services in the district and to be able to meet the needs of a broad range of women. They were prepared for their proposals to go through the standard health authority consultation procedure and to include proposals for performance monitoring of services once they were established. Their overall objectives were to establish a comprehensive therapy service for women which would augment existing and planned community mental health services. The service would include direct one-to-one work with clients, group therapy, outreach work and community development work in liaison with community mental health teams, and training for staff working in the service or seconded to it. They also identified a need to explore the possibility of establishing short term residential options for women for whom hospital admission was not considered appropriate.

The group worked for a long time. Over three years elapsed between the establishment of the group and the agreement in principle to the proposals contained in a much revised draft. During that time the draft had been circulated widely — more widely than would normally be the case for proposals relating to mental health services, and the convener of the group found herself having to respond to comments from, for example, a consultant anaesthetist and a gynaecologist. She also had to visit every planning team in the district to talk about it.

At one stage a draft was sent out to an external consultant for re writing in order to improve its acceptability. One result of that to which the group objected was the way the redraft emphasised the needs of women as carers:

> 'We feel the key point to make here is that women should not be viewed in their role as carers, but that the implications of their caring responsibilities should be considered in terms of their own health and that they should value their own health for their own sakes rather than their efficiency as carers.'

This is an example of how stereotypical assumptions about women's roles can disrupt an attempt to write women's needs into service development proposals. In this respect it is significant that one aspect of the initial draft which provoked much concern was its reference to the needs of lesbian women. It reinforces the importance of women being in a position where they are sufficiently powerful to challenge the assumptions which many in those positions hold.

The draft which was finally accepted contains most of the content of the original, a fact which owes all to the conviction and commitment of the women involved, but some sections had to be 'toned down' before they were accepted. A degree of pragmatism was felt to be vital in order to achieve their main objective of getting a strategy agreed. Once a service had been established, further developments might be possible. At the time of writing, the strategy had been accepted by the district as part of its overall community mental health strategy. But this strategy itself had not been approved by the Regional Health Authority so its future was uncertain.

The experience was in many ways a difficult one. The woman who led the task group had to find a way of building a bridge between the members of the task group who were committed to the proposals they were developing and the health authority managers and members who had to be persuaded to take the group's ideas seriously. She was in danger of losing credibility with the group if she compromised too much, and in danger of being accused of being politically naïve by senior managers if she stuck too firmly to the group's original proposals.

Stringer and Welton (1984) have written about the difficulties women in policy-making positions may experience. They identify the following risks for women in such positions:

— policy making takes a long time

— they may be 'bought off',

— there is a danger that they lose contact with other women who are disenfranchised from the policy making system,

— there tends to be a desire to formulate policy which can meet all women's needs equally and at the same time. The diverse needs of women in different situations must be recognised.

— women may experience stress as a result of working in a male-dominated system.

However, they are convinced that it is vital for women to operate at the policy level if real change is to be achieved:

Women who are in policy-making positions are professionally empowered by the system to make changes.
Through role modelling for other women and men, the
female policy-maker helps personally empower those
who see themselves as equally capable of being policy-
makers. The female-policy maker also encourages collec-
tive empowerment for women in so far as she creates
public policy that recognises women's needs as legitim-
ate. (Stringer and Welton, 1984: 48.)

Women in such positions need to develop support mechanisms
to avoid burnout. They need both to ensure their continued contact
with the women whose mental health needs they hope to meet, and
that they have personal support which reinforces their commitment
and sustains them when they feel vulnerable and under attack.
Unfortunately, that support may not be available from within the
organisation in which they work. The women we described above
made an appeal to all women whose work was concerned with
mental health in the area, not just to those within the health
authority. The identification of allies throughout the system is likely
to be an important way forward.

Ruth Popplestone's (forthcoming) study of women managers in
social services identified the need for both professional and
personal support as critical. There may not be as much recognition
of the need for support groups for those in management or
policy-making positions as there is for practitioners, but this may
be particularly important because of the separation and isolation
from other women which may be experienced in such positions.

Another way of gaining both personal support and of
strengthening the case for women's mental health to feature on the
policy agenda is to identify links with other policy areas. Most local
authorities and health authorities have equal opportunities policies
and some have women's units or positive action units. Co-operation
with those working in such units could be a source of advice about
tactics as well as of identifying ways in which mental health can be
related to other policy issues: for example, the availability of public
housing for single women or women who have left their husbands.
Other policy initiatives, anti-poverty strategies for example, may

also provide an opportunity for issues relating to women's mental health to be raised.

Building alliances is particularly important where women are very much in the minority — both as service providers and users. At Ashworth Special Hospital a working group has recently been established to look specifically at the needs of women patients. Membership is drawn from all disciplines within the hospital and from women patients. Representatives from MIND, Women in Special Hospitals (WISH) and the Mental Health Act Commission have also been invited to participate. At the same time, workers from Ashworth and Broadmoor Special Hospitals have appeared on a TV programme about the experience of women in these closed institutions, and the 1991 Biennial Report of the Mental Health Act Commission will include a section on this topic. Action on a number of fronts both provides support to those in the front line who are trying to achieve change and strengthens the possibility that change will be achieved.

Women's mental health on the agenda for action.

Any consideration of how a woman-sensitive practice can be achieved within mental health services has to respond to changes currently taking place within health and social care services. Some commentators (e.g. Wistow and Henwood, 1991) have identified opportunities as well as problems in the National Health Services and Community Care Act, 1990 which, although delayed, will provide the basis on which mental health and other community care services will be developed over the next decade. We need to consider what the opportunities might be for the development of mental health services which do not reinforce gender stereotypes and which can provide a context for the type of practice we are advocating. At the same time we need to be aware of the extent to which the proposed changes derive from ideologies which have not served women well in the past.

We can start by looking at the range of services and interventions which have been developed which women experiencing mental distress have found helpful. 'Finding our own solutions' (MIND, 1986) provides examples of a wide range of initiatives including self-help groups, women's therapy centres, accommodation projects, drop-in centres and education projects. Many of these, and others that we have mentioned in this book, have developed outside statutory service providing agencies in response to the failure of traditional social and health services as far as women are concerned. The characteristics that they have in common include: ease of access, a sharing of experiences and the aim of enabling women to take control over their own health and hence over their own lives more generally.

Another characteristic of these developments is that they break down barriers between different professionals and between professionals and the women seeking help. They acknowledge that the solutions to women's mental health difficulties must be found through addressing practical needs such as housing and money, through addressing needs for meaningful occupation, as well as providing opportunities to 'explore the contradictions in our lives' (p.7) through counselling and therapy. Sadly another feature is that the funding of many of these initiatives is often reliant on idiosyncratic decision making with a consequent risk of grants being summarily withdrawn.

One of the fundamental principles of the new world of community care is that it will be a pluralistic one. Statutory agencies have never had a monopoly on service provision and that is being formally recognised in a situation in which social services authorities will have to contract with a range of providers in order to purchase services needed.

A recognition that those seeking help should also be able to exercise choice and play a part in assessing their own needs is also included in 'Caring for People' (Secretaries of State for Health, Social Security, Wales and Scotland, 1989, para 3.2.6). The opportunity here is that care managers or those undertaking assessment of people with needs for support in the community will be more willing to look beyond their own services for help which would be appropriate for the person concerned. An increased awareness of services such as those described in the MIND publication may mean that women are put in contact with sources of support more sensitive to their needs than those which have been available from within social service departments.

Current thinking about community care generally is starting to emphasise both non-medical and non-'welfare' aspects of the needs of people with mental health problems as well as people with disabilities living in the community. An important aspect of that is a focus on employment needs. The relationship between unemployment and mental health problems has long been acknowledged (Jahoda, 1958). Employment is a key source of identity and status: it can provide the financial resources necessary to enable people to participate in the social life of the community; it can itself provide an opportunity for social contact; and it can provide the opportunity for the development of skills which can be an important source of self-esteem.

In Birmingham one of the early outcomes of the Community Care Special Action Project (CCSAP) was the development of initiatives aiming to provide more access to employment for people with special needs (see Barnes and Wistow, 1991). It is important that initiatives such as these recognise the significance of employment for women and give priority to assisting women whose self-esteem has been severely damaged by mental health problems to achieve recognition through a work role. The significance of this is clear from the words of one of the women interviewed as part of a survey commissioned by CCSAP of people with mental health problems:

> 'I started back at work two months ago . . . . its great actually . . . . I've got a very responsible job — I'm responsible for other people's lives to a certain degree . . . . I have to look after people . . . . I haven't worked for 10 years . . . . the last time I worked was before I got married . . . . I went for many interviews and I found I was getting better at being interviewed . . . . so I saw this job advertised and there were about six of us at the interview and I won it hands down apparently' (female, 30s, personality disorder). (Ritchie, Morrissey and Ward, 1988.)

The importance of regaining a role which had been the source of pride and recognition was obviously very important to Marjorie (see Chapter 5). As we commented there, she was likely to need support in her aim to go back to college to be retrained in skills which she would need to work in a contemporary office. The provision of support for women like Marjorie and like the woman quoted above should be part of a mental health practice which challenges stereotypical assumptions about women's roles. The dismissal of women's needs by disparaging references to 'neurotic housewives' must be challenged by opening up the possibilities from which women can choose in terms of the way in which they live their lives.

Part of the problem that we have identified in relation to social services work with people with mental health problems is that it has suffered because of the low priority it receives in comparison with child care work. Will a higher profile be possible if social services do not feel they have to be the service providers as well as the assessors of need? It is too early to say and it would be wrong to be too optimistic because there is concern within social services about their ability to provide an assessment of all those who would be entitled to one. However, another aspect we and others have highlighted is that there are circumstances in which mothers with mental health problems do not receive any attention in their own right, but become family 'cases' because of concern over child care.

We have suggested that some separation of responsibilities for work which focuses on the child's needs and work which addresses the mother's needs would make it easier for the woman to receive help in her own right. This may be more possible to achieve if that help comes from a separate agency from that working with the child. Part of the need may well be for advocacy in the context of child care proceedings and that must come from a separate agency. Counselling which is concerned with choices about whether continuing to be a mother to the child is in the best interests of the mother's mental health may also be more appropriate coming from someone unconnected with the child care agency.

One response to the demands placed upon social services departments by the NHS and Community Care Act has been the creation of seperate Child Care and Adult Service Divisions within some social services departments. Certainly, specialist mental health teams are becoming more common in such agencies, and fewer workers are having to weigh up the competing demands of child care and mental health cases.

Local authority social services departments were established because of a concern that welfare provision was unhelpfully split between different agencies. Their establishment has not entirely overcome difficulties arising from the fact that people's needs rarely fall comfortably within the boundaries of any one agency. Good working relationships between not only health and social services but also with education, housing and other local authority departments are vital if people's full range of needs are to be met. There are advantages to women with mental health problems in being able to turn to different sources of assistance to meet their own and their children's needs.

'Caring for People' makes explicit reference to the need to help those who care for people living in the community to limit the burden that caring may place on them. Relief of both the stress and isolation experienced by many carers could make a very positive contribution to the mental health of the women who take on this role. However, as the women we discussed above recognised, there is a danger that such support is not provided to women in their own right, but only in order that they may continue to operate in the role that is expected of them. That such a concern is well-founded is evidenced by the justification given for the support of carers in the White Paper 'Helping carers to maintain their valuable contribution to the spectrum of care is both right and a sound investment'. (HMSO, 1989: 9, para 2.3.)

Mike Fisher has considered the implications of the need to recognize the rights of carers in the context of the case management requirements of the NHS and Community Care Act (Fisher, 1990). One aspect of this, he argues, is the importance of giving a recognition of the stress of caring and offering support for that without forcing the carer to adopt the role of a client. We would go further than that and suggest that there is a need to offer support to carers separate from the care management which focuses on the person being cared for and which will continue, if that is agreed, after the death of the person cared for. Support for carers when caring stops may be even more critical in mental health terms because of the impact of bereavement, the loss of role and the adjustment that both require (see Chapter 5).

This still leaves the question of women who are neither mothers nor carers of elderly parents or others. One of us read the following among the reasons for recommending the compulsory detention of a woman in her 40s in a psychiatric hospital:

'She has no contribution to make to society.'

The woman concerned was unemployed and divorced. Her mental health problems were severe and she probably was in need of care and treatment. However, as long as psychiatrists and other mental health professionals feel such an observation has a place in recommendations for hospital admission, women cannot feel confident that their needs as individuals in their own right will get a serious consideration.

In the first chapter of this book we discussed the medical dominance of mental health services and how this influenced both the assumptions on which responses to those with mental health problems are based, as well as the way in which mental health problems are perceived both by society as a whole and by those experiencing mental distress. The new community care legislation in theory gives more acknowledgement to the role of social care agencies than there has been in the past. Social Services departments have responsibility for the only 'ring-fenced' finance which is being made available for the development of community care services. But this provision is called the 'mental illness' grant and the Department of Health's guidance on its use does little to encourage those who had hoped for some change in the balance of power between social and medical care for people with mental distress.

The grant is to be available for social care for people 'whose mental illness (including dementia, whatever its cause) is so severe that they have been accepted for treatment by the specialist psychiatric services' or in order to bring 'in touch with the specialist psychiatric services people in the community not currently in touch with those services but whose needs are so severe that it is clear that they would benefit from those services' (HC (90) 24, LAC (90) 10). Thus it is not available to provide services for those whose experiences of the specialist psychiatric services is such that they are looking for alternative forms of care. The same applies to guidance in relation to the 'Care Programme' approach which aims to ensure that there is a planned programme of care involving collaboration between different professionals in the care of people with mental health problems living in the community (HC(90) 23/HASSL(90)11).

We see little in this guidance which makes us optimistic about service developments which will be more sensitive to the needs of women and which recognise that many of those needs are not appropriately met by specialist psychiatric services. Where there are improvements we think these are more likely to come from the 'bottom up' as we have described, from groups of professionals and others working with women users to take the initiative in developing a woman-centred practice and service. Such changes may be at the margins, but can make real improvements in the lives of those women who can turn to them for help. A fundamental recasting of priorities is not going to be achieved easily and, like the women in the health authority we described above, workers committed to developing a practice more sensitive to the needs of women will have to be prepared to be pragmatic and aim for achievable change in the areas in which they have some influence, whilst being clear about how this can contribute to a longer term development of more-appropriate services.

For those continuing to work within statutory agencies, those developments will have to challenge many of the traditional ways of working which we have identified above as getting in the way of enabling a woman-sensitive practice to become a reality. A number of commentators have described the development of scientific bureaucracies in social services departments as devaluing both the skills and methods of work which women bring to social work (e.g. Howe, 1986; Hale, 1983; Dominelli and McLeod, 1989). There is a danger here of stereotyping women workers and reinforcing the view that women are naturally good at caring jobs, but not very good at being managers or planners.

Carole Sturdy, writing of her experience working in the London Women's Therapy Centre, questions whether there is any such thing as a 'feminist organisation':

> real problems involved in using the adjective 'feminist' to describe anything other than woman, or female active subjects. It is hard to see what meaning the term 'feminist' can have when used to describe an organisational structure, other than that it means that it is the sort of organisational structure which particular feminists preferred to adopt, for particular reasons at a particular point in their

history. Used in any other way, it is in danger of degener-
ating into an implicit value judgement, closing off all
discussion (Sturdy, 1987: 39).

She emphasises the importance of adopting a questioning
attitude to all organizational forms and of adopting an organisation
which is appropriate to the major task to be performed. Whilst many
radical organisations are wary of 'management', an organisation
which, like the Women's Therapy Centre now, exists mainly to
provide a service must be effectively managed. Like all agencies
faced with the problem of insufficient resources to provide the level
of service needed, the centre needs to recognise that rationing
resources involves political decisions and that such decisions have
to be publicly accounted for:

'Internal democracy and collective-working practices,
within a voluntary organisation, cannot be a substitute for
external consultation and accountability' (Sturdy, ibid:
43).

Korabik and Ayman (1989) have argued for the development of
an 'androgynous' management style so that organisations get the
best of both masculine and feminine skills without assuming that
these are necessarily associated with biological sex. One woman
manager told us how in management training in private industry the
importance of stereotypical female qualities is beginning to be
recognised although inevitably redefined in masculine terms. For
example, the formerly derided, old-style female 'butterfly brain' is
now being seen as a useful quality to deal with the demands on the
modern manager but retitled in more macho terms as 'helicopter
brain'!

We do not think it is right to imply that a concern with a high
quality service to clients is necessarily at odds with a concern to
ensure an efficiently run organisation which is capable of providing
services effectively. Social services departments and health
authorities as public services should be able to demonstrate that they
are accountable to their users and to local citizens and part of that
accountability must include an ability to demonstrate that the
services being provided are effective. The key point is the definition

of what is 'effective'. We believe that to be effective the service or care being provided should be experienced as helpful by the person receiving it.

From our conversations with women users of mental health services and from similar experiences reported elsewhere we can suggest some of the features needed in an effective mental health service for women:

— it would promote self-esteem

— it would provide care to the woman in her own right

— it would be accessible without having to leave children or have them taken into care

— it would provide space to talk through feelings and experiences in a non-threatening atmosphere

— it would provide the opportunity to meet with other women with similar experiences

— it would enable the woman to take control of her own life

— it would provide access to sources of practical help as well as to counselling, therapy and drug treatments

— it would enable the woman to receive help from a woman provider if this is her choice,

— it would acknowledge that bad feelings are common to everyone, and

— it would acknowledge the 'normality' of mental distress.

Both statutory agencies needing to demonstrate their level of performance and voluntary and private agencies entering into contracts to provide services could use these as part of a check-list against which their services should be measured. It is not the concept of performance measurement that should be considered suspect, but the way in which it is sometimes applied to judge services according to criteria which have no real meaning to those on the receiving end. The women developing the strategy for women and mental health, as described in a previous chapter said that they had built performance monitoring into their proposals not only because that was the way in which health authorities worked, but also because they saw the need to build in time and opportunity for reflection. When the demands of individual case work are high they had recognised that monitoring of work was important not only to protect the workers, but also to ensure that they were still on course in providing the kind of service which the needs of women had prompted in the first place.

Clifford *et al* (1989) have suggested that those involved in the provision of mental health services may have particular need to review the services they are providing. This is because of the tendency we have already identified to distort practice as a means of protection from the chaos represented by madness. They propose a practical system for ensuring a high quality of service which takes as its starting point the statement of the principles on which services should be based.

Elsewhere one of us has described a similar value-based approach to performance measurement (Barnes and Miller, 1988). In the context we are considering here, this would mean taking the characteristics of a woman-sensitive practice outlined above and relating these to:

1) the organisation of services
2) the content of practice
3) the characteristics and attitudes of staff providing the service
4) the opportunities for staff support and development
5) the outcomes for the women receiving the service, and
6) the perceptions of the women users about the help they had received.

The involvement of both those providing and those receiving the service in actively reviewing the way in which they work together can be an empowering process. It is based on a perception that both have responsibility for establishing ways of working which support positive mental health and it can enable both worker and user to feel more in control of the healing process.

Conclusion

Throughout this book we have tried to combine an analysis of current reality for women experiencing mental distress with suggestions for ways of developing a more-woman-sensitive practice. In this final chapter we have considered the environment into which that practice will have to fit. The analysis is rarely an optimistic one. Our proposals for change have to recognise that it takes a considerable time to alter both policy and practice when both knowledge and attitudes have to change as well. But we feel that pessimism is harmful to women whose current experience of distress demands a response now. Those engaged in training, in organisational development, in policy development and in practice all have responsibilities to draw from feminist knowledge and theory, understandings which can assist the process of developing ways of reducing that distress. For those whose power is threatened by that process it will be a painful experience. Humility in acknowledgement of the continuum of experience between 'sanity' and 'madness' for all of us may be one outcome for those prepared to open themselves up to this change.

APPENDIX

Developing a different type of practice cannot follow a blueprint. However, it is useful to have some prompts which can act as guides on the way. In this appendix we suggest some questions which we think might be helpful to those wanting to develop a mental health practice which is sensitive to the needs of women. The list is not intended to be exhaustive, but we hope those embarking on this journey may find it helpful as a means of starting to think about existing practice and of where they want to get to.

We have divided the questions under headings relating to different areas of practice, and to the organisational and policy context in which that work is carried out. However, the specific settings in which work will take place will affect the way in which questions will need to be interpreted. For example, the question: 'What is it like to be a women in her situation?' will have very different connotations when asked of a woman who has been a patient in a special hospital for many years, from those it will have if asked of a women who has become depressed and anxious following the birth of her first child. Our point is that we think it is important to understand a woman's experience of her particular situation, whatever it is, before it is possible to respond to her mental distress.

Ideally we suggest that workers should get together, perhaps with an external trainer or facilitator, and use these questions with some of the examples of women's experiences we have discussed during the course of this book, to consider how they can work together to develop a women-sensitive mental health practice.

WORK WITH INDIVIDUALS

— Have I really listened to her?

— What is it like to be a woman in her particular situation?

— What do other people around her expect from her, and is it what she wants for herself?

— What are my assumptions about the cause of her distress?

— Have I checked those out with her?

— Have I enabled her to tell me if she has been abused - as a child or more recently?

— Does she need practical support - with housing, money, help gaining employment, child care etc.?

— How can I empower her to gain support from those around her?

— Would it be useful to agree a written contract of work with her?

— Am I sure that what I think is right is meaningful for her?

GROUPWORK

— Would sharing problems with other women in similar situations help?

— Does she have the confidence to share in a group?

— Would she benefit from confidence-building to enable her to join a group?

— Would a group be less frightening than individual casework/therapy?

— Are there any circumstances in which a mixed gender group would help to address specific communication problems?

— What sort of group would be best?

— Does such a group exist or would I need to see if I could bring one together?

— Would her relationships outside the group make it difficult for her to attend?

— What sort of practical help would she need to enable her to attend?

— How would her membership of the group be likely to affect her relationships outside the group?

— Where would it be best for the group to meet?

COMMUNITY WORK

— Who are the influential people in this community who could support the development of improved facilities for women?

— How could I approach them?

— What would be my priority for action to assist the mental health of women in this community?

— What is achievable in the short term, in the long term?

— What is not achievable?

— What different communities are there in my area?

— How do I make contact with women in those different communities to identify any mental health problems and needs?

— How do I ensure that I can make contact with the most isolated women in these communities?

— How do I distinguish between general support needs and the specific mental health needs of women in these communities?

— How do I ensure that mental health needs do not get lost in responding to more general needs for community support and development?

POLICY

— Does my agency have a mental health policy which makes specific reference to the mental health needs of women?

— If so, what assumptions does it make about the origins and nature of mental distress in women?

— Does it consider the mental health needs of women of all ages, from all ethnic groups in the area and living in different family or other situations?

— Does existing policy (explicit or implicit) disadvantage women in any way?

— If we don't have a policy, what can I do to ensure that one is developed?

— Whom do I need to work with in order to do this? Are there pressure groups/allies already available or will I have to develop these?

— What research is available that would help in formulating a policy?

— What knowledge or expertise is there amongst people working with women in this area?

— How can I enable women users of mental health services to make an input to developing a policy?

— Are there other areas of policy which would be worth making links with?

— How will we know if the policy has been implemented successfully?

THE WORKER IN THE ORGANISATION

— How can I find ways of looking at my own prejudices and assumptions?

— Whom do I need as an ally to support my feminist practice?

— Where is my support group?

— How do working practices within my organisation challenge or reinforce the approach I am trying to develop?

— Are there aspects of working practice which I will need to try to change to enable me to implement a feminist practice?

— How do I deal with the tension between what I want to achieve with women experiencing mental distress and the current reality of their lives?

— How do I acknowledge and deal with my own mental distress?

— How do I protect my own mental health?

BIBLIOGRAPHY

ADSS West Midlands Region. (1989) *Social Services Support to People with a Mental Health Problem. A Collaborative Approach.*

Bailey, S. (1987) A Mental Health Centre: the Users' View in its Evaluation. *Social Services Research, (3)*: 25–8.

Baker, A.W. and Duncan, S.P. (1985) Child Sexual Abuse: a Study of Prevalence in Great Britain, *Child Abuse and Neglect*, 9: 457–67.

Banton, R. Clifford, P. Frosh, S. Lousada, J. and Rosenthall, J. (1985) *The Politics of Mental Health.* Basingstoke, Macmillan.

Barnes, M. and Miller, N. (1988) Performance Measurement in Personal Social Services, *Research, Policy and Planning*, 6: 2.

Barnes , M. and Prior, D. (1984) *Monitoring the Impact of the Mental Health Act 1983,* London Borough of Hounslow Social Services Department.

Barnes, M. Bowl, R. and Fisher, M. (1990) *Sectioned: Social Services and the 1983 Mental Health Act.* London, Routledge.

Barnes, M. and Wistow, G. (1991) *Changing Relationships in Community Care; an interim account of the Birmingham Community Care Special Action Project,* Nuffield Institute for Health Service Studies, University of Leeds.

Barnes, M. et al (1986) *Monitoring The Mental Health Act 1983. A Report of the Collaborative Project,* University of Birmingham, Social Services Research Group.

Barrett, M. and McIntosh, M. (1982) *The Anti-Social Family.* London, Verso.

171

Baruch, E.H. and Sevanno, L.J. (1988) *Women Analyse Women*, New York, New York University Press.

Bernal, J. and Dalton, J. (1990) A Women's Support Group, *Royal College of Psychiatrists Bulletin*, 14: 9, 531–33.

Bettelheim, B. (1987) *A Good Enough Parent*, London, Thames and Hudson.

Bowl, R. (1986) Social Work with Old People, in C. Phillipson and A. Walker (eds), *Ageing and Social Policy: a Critical Assessment*, Aldershot, Gower.

Bowlby, J. (1980) *Attachment and Loss: Loss, Sadness and Depression* (vol iii) New York, Basic Books.

Brandt, L.M. (1989) A Short-term Group Therapy Model for Treatment of Adult Female Survivors of Childhood Incest, *Group*, 13: 2, 74–82.

Briere, J. (1984) *The Effects of Childhood Abuse on Later Psychological Functioning; Defining a Post-Sexual Abuse Syndrome*, Paper presented at 3rd National Conference on Sexual Victimisation of Children. Washington, D.C., Children's Hospital National Medical Centre.

Brook, E. and Davis, A. (1985) (eds), *Women, The Family and Social Work*. London, Tavistock.

Broverman, D., Clarkson, F., Rosenkrantz, P., Vogel, S. and Broverman, I. (1970) Sex-role stereotype and clinical judgements of mental health, *Journal of Consulting and Clinical Psychology*, 34: 1–7.

Brown, G. and Harris, T. (1978) *Social Origins of Depression: A Study of Psychiatric Disorder in Women*. London, Tavistock.

Brown, G W., Craig, T K J. and Harris, T.O. (1985) Depression: distress or disease? Some Eepidemiological Cconsiderations. *British Journal of Psychiatry*, 147: 612–22.

Butler, A. and Pritchard, C. (1983) *Social Work and Mental Illness*, London, Macmillan.

Butler, S. and Wintram, C. (1991) *Feminist Groupwork*, London, Sage.

Cain, M. (ed), (1989) *Growing Up Good. Policing the Behaviour of Girls in Europe*. London, Sage.

Campbell, B. (1988) *Unofficial Secrets. Child Sexual Abuse: the Cleveland Case*. London, Virago.

Campbell, P. (1990) Self-Harm, *Openmind*, 42: 17.

Cantley, C. (1990) Crisis Intervention: Users' Views of a Community Mental Health Service, *Research, Policy and Planning*, 8: 1, 1–6.

Casement (1985) *On Learning from the Patient*, London & New York, Tavistock.

Chambless, D.L. and Goldstein, A.J. (1980) Anxieties: Agoraphobia and Hysteria, in A M Brodsky and R Hare-Mustin (eds), *Women and Psychotherapy*, New York, The Guildford Press.

Chodoff, P. (1982) Hysteria and Women, *American Journal of Psychiatry*, 139: 545–51.

Chodorow, N. (1978) *The Reproduction of Mothering: Psychoanalysis and the sociology of gender*, Berkeley, University of California Press.

Clifford, P., Leiper, R., Lavender, A. and Pilling, S. (1989) *Assuring Quality in Mental Health Services*, London, RDP in association with Free Association Books.

Cochrane, R. (1983) *The Social Creation of Mental Illness*, London, Longman.

Cohen, J. and Fisher, M. (1987) Recognition of Mental Health Problems by Doctors and Social Workers. *Practice*, 1 (3): 225–40.

Connelly, N. (1990) *Raising Voices: Social Services Departments and People with Disabilities*, London, Policy Studies Institute.

Corob, A. (1987) *Working with Depressed Women* Aldershot, Gower.

Crawley, C. (1988): Feminism and the Older Woman - An Area of Neglect. *Action Baseline*, Autumn, 7–12.

Croft, S. and Beresford, P. (1990) *From Paternalism to Participation; involving people in social services*, London, Open Services Project and Joseph Rowntree Foundation.

Crossroads Care (1990) *A Profile of Carers: Commentary*.

Curran, V. and Golombok, S. (1985) *Bottling it Up*, London, Faber and Faber.

Dale, J. and Foster, P. (1986) *Feminists and State Welfare*, London, Routledge and Kegan Paul.

Department of Health and Welsh Office (1990) *Code of Practice;* laid before Parliament in December 1989 pursuant to section 118(4) of the Mental Health Act 1983, London, HMSO.

Dohrenwend, B.P. (1973) Life Events as Stressors: a Methodological Enquiry, *Journal of Health and Social Behaviour*, 14: 167–175.

Dohrenwend, B.P. and Dohrenwend, B.S. (eds) (1974), *Stressful Life Events: Their Nature and Effects*, New York, John Wiley.

Dominelli, L. and McLeod, E. (1989) *Feminist Social Work*, Basingstoke, Macmillan.

Ehrenreich, B. and English, D. (1979) *For Her Own Good. 150 Years of the Experts' Advice to Women.* London, Pluto Press.

Emerson, R. and Pollner, M. (1975) Dirty Work Designations; their Features and Consequences in a psychiatric setting, *Social Problems*, 23: 243–54.

Erikson, E.H. (1963) *Childhood and Society,* New York, Norton.

Ernst, S. (1987) Can a Daughter be a Woman? in S. Ernst and M. Maguire (eds), *Living with the Sphinx*, London, The Women's Press.

Ernst, S. and Goodison, L. (1981) *In Our Own Hands*, London, The Women's Press.

Ernst, S. and Maguire, M. (eds), (1987) *Living with the Sphinx*, London, The Women's Press.

Ernst, S. (1989) Gender and the Phantasy of Omnipotence: Case Study of an Organisation, in Richards, B. (ed), *Crises of the Self,* London, Free Association Books.

Evans, N., Kendall, I., Lovelock, R. and Powell, J. (1986) *Something to Look Forward To: an Evaluation of a Travelling Day Hospital for Elderly People,* Portsmouth Polytechnic, Social Services Research and Intelligence Unit.

Fabrikant, B. (1974) The Psychotherapist and the Female Patient: Perceptions and Change, in V. Franks and V. Burtle (eds), *Women in Therapy,* New York: Bruner/Mazel.

Finch, J. and Groves, D. (1985) Old Girl, Old Boy: Gender Divisions in Social Work with the Elderly, in E Brook and A Davis (eds), *Women, The Family and Social Work,* London, Tavistock.

Fisher, M., Newton C., and Sainsbury, E. (1984) *Mental Health Social Work Observed.* London, George Allen and Unwin.

Foulkes (1964) *Therapeutic Group Analysis*, London, Maresfield.

Fransella, F. and Frost, K. (1977) *On Being a Woman*, London, Tavistock.

Freud, S. (1977) Female Sexuality (1931), in *The Penguin Freud 7 On Sexuality*, Harmondsworth, Penguin.

Furniss, T., Bingley-Miller, L., and Van Elburg, A. (1988) Goal-oriented Group Treatment for Sexually Abused Adolescent Girls, *British Journal of Psychiatry*, 152: 97–106.

Garside, R F., Kay, D W K., and Roth, M. (1965) Old Age and Mental Disorders in Newcastle-upon-Tyne, *British Journal of Psychiatry*, 111: 939–946.

Gelsthorpe, L. (1985) Normal, natural trouble: girls and juvenile justice, *Lay Panel Magazine* (Northern Ireland Courts Association, Belfast), pp.1–9.

Gilleard, C. (1985) The Psychogeriatric Patient and the Family, in G. Horobin (ed) *Responding to Mental Illness, Research Highlights in Social Work*, 11, London, Kogan Page.

Goldberg, D. and Huxley, P. (1980) *Mental Illness in the Community*. London, Tavistock.

Goldner, V. (1985) Feminism and Family Therapy, *Family Process*, 24: 1; 33–47.

Gottesman, I.I. and Shields, J. (1982) *Schizophrenia; The Epigenetic Puzzle*, Cambridge, Cambridge University Press.

Grabucker, M. (1988) *There's a Good Girl*, London, The Women's Press.

Gray, B. and Isaacs, B. (1979) *Care of the Elderly Mentally Infirm*, London, Tavistock.

Gray, T. and Swindell, L. (1987) *Young women's sexual abuse group-evaluation report*, Greenwich Social Services, Thamesmead Family Services Unit.

Greenspan, M. (1983) *A New Approach to Women and Therapy*, McGraw-Hill.

Hale, J. (1983) Feminism and Social Work Practice, in B. Jordan and N. Parton (eds), *The Political Dimensions of Social Work*, Oxford, Basil Blackwell.

Hare-Mustin, R. (1987) The Problem of Gender in *Family Therapy*, *Family Process*, 26: 15–27.

Hartman, A. (1989) Growing up Female: a Different Route, *Smith College Studies in Social Work: Special Issue — Women and Clinical Practice*, 59: 3, 252–265.

Hirsch, S.R. and Leff, J.P. (1975) *Abnormalities in parents of schizophrenics*, Institute of Psychiatry, Maudsley Monograph, London, OUP.

Hite, S. (1990) 'I Hope I'm Not Like Mother' in J. Price Knowles and E. Cole (eds) *Woman Defined Motherhood*, New York, Harrington Park Press.

Holmes, T.H. and Rahe, R.H. (1967) The Social Readjustment Rating scale, *Journal of Psychosomatic Research*, 11: 213–18.

Hooyman, N.R. (1987) Older Women and Social Work Curricula, in D. Burden and N. Gottlieb (eds), *The Woman Client*, New York and London, Tavistock Publications.

Hoppe, R.B. (1985) The Case For or Against Diagnostic and Therapeutic Sexism, in C.T. Mowbray *et al* (eds). *Women and Mental Health — New Directions for Change*, New York, Harrington Park Press.

Horizon, (1989) *Newpin — A Lifeline,* Script of the programme transmitted 19.6 and 20.6. London, BBC Publications.

Howe, D. (1986) The Segregation of Women and Their Work in the Personal Social Services, *Critical Social Policy,* 15; 21–36.

Hudson, A. (1988) Boys will be Boys: Masculinism and the Juvenile Justice System, *Critical Social Policy,* 21 (Spring): 30–48.

Hudson, A. (1989) 'Troublesome Girls' Towards Alternative Definitions and Policies, in M. Cain (ed) *Growing up Good. Policing the behaviour of girls in Europe.* London, Sage.

Hudson, B. (1989) Decision Making about Girls within the Criminal Justice System, in M. Cain (ed), *Growing Up Good. Policing the behaviour of girls in Europe.* London, Sage.

Hudson, B. (1982) *Social Work with Psychiatric Patients,* London, Macmillan.

Hunt, A. (1978) *The Elderly at Home,* London, HMSO.

Hunter, J. (1985) Aged People in a Short Term Therapeutic Group, *Journal of Social Work Practice,* 1: 4, 49–65.

Hunter, J. (1989) Age Old Feelings, *Openmind,* no. 39: 12–13.

Hutchings, S. (1989) Sectioning — A Last Resort, *Openmind,* 40: 11.

Ineichen, B., Harrison, G. and Morgan, H.G. (1984) Psychiatric Hospital Admissions in Bristol, I, geographical or ethnic factors, *British Journal of Psychiatry,* 150: 505–512.

Jahoda, M. (1958) *Current Concepts of Positive Mental Health,* New York, Basic Books.

Jenkins, R. (1985) Sex Differences in Minor Psychiatric Morbidity: a Survey of a Homogeneous Population, *Social Science and Medicine*, 20: 9, 887–899.

Jenner, A. (1988) A Psychiatrist's Apologia, in *Report of Common Concerns; International conference on user involvement in mental health services*, East Sussex CC, Brighton Health Authority, MIND.

Jervis, M. (1991) Grey Area, *Social Work Today*, 11.4.

Jones, L. and Cochrane, R. (1981) Stereotypes of Mental Illness: a Test of the Labelling Hypothesis, *International Journal of Social Psychiatry*, 27: 99–107.

Jowell, R., Witherspoon, S. and Brook, L. (eds), (1989) *British Social Attitudes: Special International Report* , London, Gower.

Jowell, R., Witherspoon, S. and Brook, L. (eds), (1988) *British Social Attitudes, the 5th Report*, Aldershot, Gower/SCPR.

Kaplan, A.G. and Surrey, J.L. (1986) The Relational Self in Women: Developmental Theory and Public Policy, in L E Walker, (ed), *Women and Mental Health Policy*, Beverly Hills and London, Sage Publications.

Korabik, K. and Ayman, R. (1989) Do Women Managers Have to Act Like Men? *The Journal of Management Development*, 8: 6, 23–32.

Kubler-Ross, E. (1969) *On Death and Dying*. New York, Macmillan.

Lawrence, M. and Dana, M. (1990) *Fighting Food*, Harmondsworth, Penguin.

Lazare, A. and Klerman, G. L. (1968) Hysteria and Depression: the Frequency and Significance of Hysterical Personality Features in Hospitalised Depressed Women, *American Journal of Psychiatry*, 124: 48–56.

Lees, S. (1989) The Policing of Girls in Everyday Life, in M. Cain (ed) *Growing Up Good. Policing the behaviour of girls in Europe*. London, Sage.

Levine, S. (1986) *Who Dies: An investigation of conscious living and conscious dying*. Bath, Gateway Books.

Linn M.W., Hunter, K.I. and Perry, P.R. (1979) Differences by Sex and Ethnicity in the Psychosocial Adjustment of the Elderly, *Journal of Health and Social Behaviour*, 20: 273-281.

MacIntyre, S. and Oldman, D. (1977) Coping with Migraine, in A. Davis and G. Horobin (eds) *Medical Encounters*, London, Croom Helm.

MacLeod, S. (1981) *The Art of Starvation*, London, Virago.

Maple, N.A. (1984) *A Study of the Role of Crisis Intervention Strategies in the Psychiatric Emergency, with Particular Reference to Current Social Work Practice in an Outer London Borough*, unpub M Soc Sc dissertation.

Maple, N.A. (1988) Cognitive Analytic Therapy as Part of the Social Work Service provided by a Social Services Area Team, *Social Services Research*, (2): 18–29.

McCormick, E.W.(1988) *Nervous Breakdown*, London, Unwin.

Mednick, S. A., Schulsinger, F. and Venables, P.H. (1981) A Fifteen-year Follow-up of Children with Schizophrenic Mothers (Denmark) in S. A. Mednick and A. E.Baert (eds), *Prospective Longitudinal Research: An Empirical Basis for the Primary Prevention of Psychosocial Disorders*, Oxford, Oxford University Press on behalf of WHO Regional Office for Europe.

Menzies, I.E.P. (1961) *The Functioning of Social Systems as a Defence Against Anxiety*, Pamphlet no 3, London, Tavistock.

Miller, A. (1987) *For Your Own Good*, London, Virago.

Miller, A. (1984) *Thou Shalt Not Be Aware: Society's Betrayal of the Child*, London, Virago. Miller, J.B. (1988) Toward a New Psychology of Women, Harmondsworth, Penguin.

MIND (1986) *Finding Our Own Solutions; Women's Experience of Mental Health Care*, London MIND Publications.

Mitchell, J. (1974) *Psychoanalysis and Feminism*, Harmondsworth, Penguin.

Morgan, H.G., Purgold, J. and Welbourne, J. (1983) Management and Outcome in Anorexia Nervosa: a Standardised Prognosis Study, *British Journal of Psychiatry*, 143: 282-287.

Murphy, E. (1982) Social Origins of Depression in Old Age, *British Journal of Psychiatry*, 141: 135-142.

Nairne, K. and Smith, G. (1984) *Dealing with Depression*, London, The Women's Press.

Newson, J. and Newson, E. (1976) Day to Day Aggression between Parent and Child, in N. Tutt (ed), *Violence in London*, London, DHSS/HMSO.

Newton, J. (1988) *Preventing Mental Illness*, London, Routledge.

Oakley, A. (1980) *Women Confined. Towards a Sociology of Childbirth*. Oxford, Martin Robertson.

Olivier, C. (1989) *Jocasta's Children, The Imprint of the Mother*, London, Routledge.

Orbach, S. (1978) *Fat is a Feminist Issue*, London, Hamlyn.

Pallot, P. (1991) Nurse Doubles Her Age to Prove a Point, *Daily Telegraph, 1*8th August.

Parry-Crooke, G. and Ryan, J. (1986) *Evaluation of Self-Help Groups for Women with Compulsive Eating Problems,* London, Health Education Authority.

Peace, S. (1986) The Forgotten Female, in C. Phillipson and A. Walker (eds), *Ageing and Social Policy: a Critical Assessment*, Aldershot, Gower.

Policy Studies Institute (1990) *Credit and Debt in Britain*, London, PSI.

Popplestone, R. (forthcoming) Women Managers — Finding an Easier Route up the Ladder, *Social Services Research.*

Pound, A. and Mills, M. (1983) *The Impact of Maternal Depression on Young Children,* Paper presented at the Tavistock Centre Scientific Meeting.

Pound, A., Mills, M., and Cox T. (1985) A Pilot Evaluation of Newpin, a Homevisiting and Befriending Scheme in South London, October *Newsletter of the Association of Child Psychology and Psychiatry.*

Price, J. (1988) *Motherhood, What it Does to Your Mind,* London, Pandora Press.

Rich, A. (1977) *Of Woman Born; Motherhood as Experience and Institution,* London, Virago.

Ritchie, J., Morrissey, C. and Ward, K. (1988) *Keeping in Touch with the Talking; The Community Care Needs of People with Mental Illness,* Birmingham, Community Care Special Action Project/Social and Community Planning Research.

Robertson, J. (1983) Menopause, *Spare Rib*, 127; 50–55.

Rogers, A. and Faulkner, A. (1987) *A Place of Safety*, London, MIND.

Rosenkrantz, P., Vogel, S., Bee, H., Broverman, I. and Broverman, D. (1968) Sex-role Stereotypes and Self-concepts in College Students, *Journal of Consulting and Clinical Psychology*, 32: 287–95.

Rosenthall, J. and Greally, B. (1988) *Women and Depression*, London, Islington Women and Mental Health.

Roth, R. and Lerner, J. (1974) Sex-based Discrimination in the Mental Institutionalisation of Women, *California Law Review*, 62: 789–815.

Russo, N.F. (1984) Women in the Mental Health Delivery System: Implications for Research and Public Policy, in L.E. Walker (ed), *Women and Mental Health Policy*, Beverly Hills and London, Sage Publications.

Rutter, M. (1971) Parent-child Separation: Psychological Effects on Children, *Jnl of Child Psychology and Psychiatry, 12*: 233–260.

Rycroft, C. (1979) *A Critical Dictionary of Psychoanalysis*, Harmondsworth, Penguin Books.

Ryle, A. (1990) *Cognitive Analytic Therapy: Active Participation in Change*, Chichester, Wiley.

Satyamurti, C. (1979) Care and Control in Local Authority Social Work, in N. Parry., M Rustin. and C. Satyamurti (eds), *Social Work, Welfare and the State*, London, Edward Arnold.

Secretaries of State for Health, Social Security, Wales and Scotland (1989) *Caring for People: Community Care in the Next Decade and Beyond*, CM 849, London, HMSO.

Seligman, M.E.P. (1975) *Helplessness: On Depression, Development and Death*, San Francisco, W H Freeman.

Sheldon, H. (1988) Childhood Sexual Abuse in Adult Female Psychotherapy Referrals, *British Journal of Psychiatry*, 152: 107–111.

Sheppard, M. (1990) *Mental Health: The Role of the Approved Social Worker*, Joint Unit for Social Services Research, University of Sheffield/Community Care.

Showalter, E. (1987) *The Female Malady, Women, Madness and English Culture 1830-1980*, London, Virago.

Siegel, R.J. (1990) Old Women as Mother Figures, in J. Price-Knowles and E. Cole (eds), *Woman Defined Motherhood*, New York, Harrington Park Press.

Smith, R. and Newman, E. (1982) *Self-Esteem in the Elderly*, Unpublished project report, London Borough of Hounslow Social Services Department.

Stephenson, P. (1989) Women in Special Hospitals, *Openmind*, 41, Oct/Nov: 14–16.

Stringer, D.M. and Welton, N.R. (1984) Female Psychologists in Policymaking Positions, in L.E. Walker (ed), *Women and Mental Health Policy*, vol 9 Sage Yearbooks in Women's Policy Studies, Beverly Hills and London, Sage Publication.

Sturdy, C. (1987) Questioning the Sphinx: an Experience of Working in a Women's Organisation, in S. Ernst and M. Maguire (eds), *Living with the Sphinx*, London, Women's Press.

Swindell, L. (forthcoming) Working with Care and Authority: a Groupwork Approach to Child Sexual Abuse, in M. Whitfield (ed), *Child Sexual Abuse (provisional title)*, Family Services Units, 207 Old Marylebone Road, London NW1 5QP, due for publication Spring 1992.

Szmuckler, G.I., Bird, A.S. and Button, E.J. (1981) Compulsory Admissions in a London Borough: I Social and Clinical Features and Follow-up, *Psychological Medicine*, 11: 617–36.

Theander, S. (1985) Outcome and Prognosis in Anorexia Nervosa and Bulimia: Some Results of Previous Investigations Compared with those of a Swedish Long-term Study, *Journal of Psychiatric Research 19*, 493–508.

Townsend, P. (1979) *Poverty in the United Kingdom*, Harmondsworth, Penguin.

Treasure, J. (1991) Long-term Management of Eating Disorders, *International Journal of Psychiatry*, 3, 43–58.

Twigg, J., Atkin, K. and Perring, C. (1990) *Carers and Services: A Review of Research*, London, HMSO.

Ungerson, C. (1987) *Policy is Personal; Sex, Gender and Informal Care*, London, Tavistock.

Vaughn, C.E. and Leff, J.P. (1976) The Influence of Family and Social Factors on the Course of Psychiatric Illness: a Comparison of Schizophrenic and Depressed Neurotic Patients, *British Journal of Psychiatry* 129, 125–37.

Veith, I. (1965) *Hysteria: The History of a Disease*, University of Chicago Press.

Warner, A. (1987) The Quality of Life for Elderly People Living in Birmingham's Residential Homes, *Social Services Research*, 3: 11–23.

Welburn, V. (1980) *Postnatal Depression*, Glasgow, Fontana.

Wilkin, D. and Hughes, B. (1986) The Elderly and the Health Services, in C. Phillipson and A. Walker (eds), *Ageing and Social Policy: a Critical Assessment*, Aldershot, Gower.

Winokur, G. and Leonard, C. (1963) Sexual Life in Patients with Hysteria, *Diseases of the Nervous System,* 24: 337–343.

Wistow, G. and Henwood, M. (1991) Caring for People: Elegant Model or Flawed Design? in N. Manning (ed), *Social Policy Review 1990/91,* London, Longman.

Index